Sexual Liberation or Sexual License?

SEXUAL LIBERATION OR SEXUAL LICENSE?

*The American Revolt
Against Victorianism*

Kevin White

The American Ways Series

IVAN R. DEE   *Chicago*

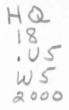

HQ
18
.U5
W5
2000

Library of Congress Cataloging-in-Publication Data:
White, Kevin, 1959–
    Sexual liberation or sexual license? : the American revolt against
Victorianism / Kevin White.
        p.   cm. — (The American ways series)
    Includes bibliographical references and index.
    ISBN 1-56663-305-2 (cloth : alk. paper) — ISBN 1-56663-306-0
(paper : alk. paper)
    1. Sex customs—United States—History.   I. Title.   II. Series.
HQ18.U5 W5 2000
306.7'0973—dc21   00-023764

In memory of Jeff

Contents

Acknowledgments

I would like to thank John Braeman and Ivan Dee for giving me the opportunity to write this book, and for their heroic patience. The staff of the University of Sussex and Portsmouth libraries have been particularly supportive, and the staff of the Library of Congress have been, as ever, great at locating sources. Several relatives and friends and colleagues have helped me in recent years—David Barry, Julia Courtney, Ray Douglas, Michael Dunne, James Dye, Rick Edgar, Paula and Hervé Graulle, Stuart Hobbs, Sharon MacManus, Sara McClachlan, Randolf Reder, Colin and Mary White. And Hélène. Leila Rupp and John Burnham have continued to be inspirations after twenty years. In the very final stages, Graham Hodges and the 1999 Colgate University London Study Group reminded me again of the pleasure of teaching American undergraduates. I hope the stimulation they gave me shows in the pages that follow.

K. W.

Worthing, West Sussex
April 2000

Sexual Liberation or Sexual License?

1

Victorian America

DESCRIBING CULTURE in the United States between 1830 and 1910, historians usually refer to "Victorian America." This is not homage to the great British queen empress. Nor is it in deference to British world dominance, for by the end of the century the United States had firmly found its feet internationally. Rather it indicates that American culture was still an extension of the British, and that after 1830 both the British middle class and the British-American ethnic group that dominated the United States accepted what have come to be known popularly as "Victorian values."

Victorian values have become linked in people's minds with sexual repression and prudery. Indeed, until the mid-1970s, historians suggested that Victorians deliberately tried to blot out everything that suggested sex. The most notorious example appeared in an 1837 travel book by the English children's writer Captain Marryat, who observed that in New England the legs of tables were covered with little breeches "lest they suggest the female limb." Further, at dinner it was thought to be good manners to say "Pass the chicken bosoms," not "breasts," because "breasts" was seen as too daring a word. No wonder Victorians were not supposed to take their clothes off to have sex and English mothers admonished their daughters to "lie down and think of England" on their wedding night.

Victorian morality was, according to this view, the morality of Puritans and of prudish, interfering "Mrs. Grundys" (a famously prudish character from an early English novel, *Speed the Plough*).

But there are many reasons to suspect that American ideas were typical of the Victorians. Here was the freest country the world had ever seen. Its experiment in democracy was proving remarkably durable, and foreign observers like the Frenchman Alexis de Tocqueville already had noted that its men and women were moving toward greater equality with each other. Young women in the United States, Tocqueville said, enjoyed greater freedom before marriage than in any other country. Could it be that such a strong control over people's personal lives could exist in a society that was so decentralized? And, surely, didn't some men and women enjoy sex? The sense of the forbidden alone should have made it seem all the more exciting. It seems naive to imagine that natural pleasure should be curtailed in a land whose frontier spirit demanded a practical attitude toward sexual relations. Something has seemed profoundly wrong with what the philosopher Michel Foucault has called the "repressive hypothesis" of Victorianism.

At the same time there is no question that the Victorians lived in a world very different from ours. Victorians believed that a healthy society could not survive without the control of instincts. This was the linchpin of a rigorous public morality. The great Irish orator and parliamentarian Edmund Burke influenced Victorian thinking: "Men are qualified for civil liberty in exact proportion to their disposition to put moral chains upon their own appetites. . . . Society cannot exist unless a controlling power upon will and appetite be placed somewhere, and the less of it there is within, the more there must be without." This was not a morality that was to be imposed by force. Because it was the morality of "civil society," it depended on the strength of neighborly familial authority and the regard of a younger generation for its elders.

The historian Gertrude Himmelfarb has suggested that this control of instincts was maintained not by means of a set of "values" but rather by a tally of "virtues." These were not the classical or Christian virtues. Nor did most Victorians understand them as anything quite so crass as Benjamin Franklin's "twelve virtues" as they appeared in his *Autobiography,* and which every American schoolboy would have read: "Trust not to venality except for health." Rather they involved "a sense of gravity and authority" that was shared by everyone. In a society that focused on the production of goods and was on the verge of an industrial leap, certain of these "virtues" were thought to be essential to survival: thrift, self-sacrifice, self-help, hard work, responsibility, honesty, persistence. These were qualities that promised rewards down the line rather than in the present.

Above all, to possess these "virtues" assured "respectability." This word did not have the suggestion of conformist mediocrity that our age has bestowed on it. Rather, in the nineteenth-century American context, it described a man or woman who possessed "character," who embodied all the key virtues. In short, "character" stood for the main qualities of the American "New Man" or "New Adam." The idea was profoundly democratic because anyone, man or woman, could attain character. It was a middle-class ethos, yet its influence extended upward to the upper class and downward to the working class. No question that Victorian America was a demanding society in which to live. We cannot therefore expect Victorians to share our view that morals are relative; Victorians thought in absolutes. The expected standard was not one of many alternatives but one of appropriate behavior. If taboos were broken, sanctions could be imposed.

The character of a man or woman depended on his or her

conduct of family and personal life. A man's character was revealed by how he treated women. To be truly manly, Victorian males had to be gentlemen. A gentleman should control his primitive urges. Marriage manuals encouraged males to be "athletes of continence." As one writer put the matter, "man's pivotal passion is the sexual." Another warned that men "love lust for lust's sake." Therefore "indulgence inflames . . . the more it is indulged, the more it demands." Male sexuality needed to be both controlled and refined so that a gentleman respected women. American men took pride in that, as Mark Twain explained, "a lady may traverse our states all day, going and coming as she chooses and never be molested by any man." This suggested the superiority of the new American man to the European. Twain wrote with utter contempt of the Englishman Colonel Valentine Baker who had harassed some women in a railway carriage. To Victorians, a rapist was the lowest of men. Gentlemen who could not control their primitive urges and instincts threatened the social equilibrium. Thus many Victorians insisted on purity before marriage as a safeguard. Theodore Roosevelt on his wedding night wrote in his diary "Thank God I am perfectly pure." Not every writer was as firm as health faddist Sylvester Graham, who argued that sperm was like a lifeblood for men and should not be wasted. Later in the century, in 1897, the author of *What a Young Man Ought to Know* linked the spending of semen with "self-pollution," which could entail "evil thoughts," the examining of "nude and nasty" pictures, masturbation, or "illicit" sex, which meant sex before marriage. Marriage manuals, while they were euphemistic about sex, were obsessed with the dangers of masturbation, "the solitary vice." Sex itself was described by one writer as an "unfortunate necessity."

This focus on continence and chastity in public pronouncements on virtue drew further strength from the "conspiracy of silence" about sexuality. Discussion of sex might incite excessive curiosity about the subject. Later generations have considered this a sign of prudery. Not so. The historian Karen Lystra has recently shown how "public reticence was a sign of good breeding." Americans were therefore serious about their application of the conspiracy right up to the turn of the century. When in 1899 an eminent Chicago physician tried to discuss "the hygiene of the sexual act" at a meeting of the American Medical Association, he was not permitted to do so. A Baltimore gynecologist protested that "discussion of the subject is attended with filth and we besmirch ourselves by discussing it in public." This was not squeamishness on the doctor's part but simply the expected behavior of a man of character. When the Reverend Phillip Moxon spoke in the year 1890 to a YMCA meeting about the subject of sex, he proclaimed that "this subject is not of my choosing, save as to the form in which it is put. . . . How shall I fitly and plainly say what needs to be said without revolting those who hear from a subject which every one of us would gladly drop into oblivion?" A gentleman simply did not talk about sex in public in Victorian America.

And a lady certainly did not. In their public pronouncements, Victorians preferred to deny the very existence of female sexuality. They expected women to conform to the "cult of true womanhood," that is, to be "pious, pure, domesticated, and submissive." Women were segregated into the private sphere, quite separate from the public world of men. They should be "passionless" too, in bed. According to this common nineteenth-century idea, women were "angels," up on a pedestal and revered as being above carnal and earthly things. The historian Nancy Cott has suggested that "the positive contribution of passionlessness was to replace that sexual/carnal characterization of women with a spiritual/moral one." On the one hand, women could assert control in the sexual sphere; on the other, "passionlessness" meant a denial that

women had erotic feelings. For a woman of character, however, "passionlessness" was the guide to best conduct. Women
were the very upholders of the moral order; their responsibility was to tame the rampant sexuality of men. A vast literature
appeared on "the lack of female sexuality." Although most of
these writers did not go as far as to declare that women's sexuality was physiologically weaker than that of men, all accepted
it was different from men's and on a higher plane. Public ideas
about women's sexuality therefore aimed at preserving propriety.

How far did these lofty standards of the public world re-
flect real lived experience? The writer Henry Seidl Canby, in
a 1934 *Harper's* memoir of courtship in the 1890s, noted that
his generation saw themselves as "gentlemen who lived by
honor." The journalist Walter Lippmann recalled that the
"virtuous man, by popular standards, was one who before his
marriage did not have sexual relations with a virtuous
woman." A young man, if he was frequently received at a
young lady's, knew that he had her favor and, above all, the
approval of the other female members of her family. Should
the young couple choose to go out, the young lady's family ensured that a third party or chaperone accompanied them. This
worked because it made certain that men as well as women
had to maintain their reputations. The humorist James
Thurber's mother remembered that in Ohio in the 1890s "you
didn't dare walk with a man after sunset, unless he was your
husband, and even then there was talk." An old man who was
interviewed for the pioneering sociological study of Muncie,
Indiana (*Middletown*), in the 1920s, recalled that "the fellows
nowadays don't seem to mind being seen on the street with a
fast woman, but you bet we did then." Hence the rituals of
courtship enforced the sturdy Victorian moral code of character.

These examples suggest the popular image of Victorian sexual morality. But within limits Victorians also gave free rein to young people. Victorians did not disparage sex; they protected it. They gave young people the privacy in which love could flourish. As a couple got to know each other and developed a relationship, they could spend time alone. As they grew closer to engagement, a couple could develop a physical intimacy. They might kiss. They might pet. They might even, once engaged, have full sexual intercourse. All of this was permissible within the moral code of the private sphere. For Victorians did not worry so much about what a young couple did; they were more concerned about the attitude of mind with which they did it. The public and private spheres blended together in high-mindedness and high standards. Americans considered it essential that young people treat one another with attitudes consistent with the idea of character.

Above all they should respect one another's manhood and womanhood by cultivating "romantic love," an idea that had been gaining ground over two centuries. As the European middle classes seized the social initiative from the aristocracy, they no longer arranged marriages but instead chose their own partners. In Europe the family and the church continued to play an enormous role in determining choice of mate until the nineteenth century. But in the United States, a far frontier of Western civilization, both church and family had always been relatively weak. By 1830 young men and women enjoyed unusual freedom in choosing a mate. Indeed Henry Seidl Canby recalled the era as "a golden age of companionship for youth." Hence "romantic love" became the main means of ensuring that free young men and women respected each other. As a well-known humorist of the time noted: "The sexes have learned to cultivate the proper degree of delicacy in their intercourse." In a culture steeped in Christian imagery, yet one in which Christianity was steadily losing its grip on people, romantic love became a key focus of young men and women's hopes for emotional fulfillment. If people lacked the faith that happiness, if not attainable here, could be gained in the next life, they tried all the more to ensure that they would achieve it in this world.

It should not surprise us that romantic love became infused with religious language. Being in love was like being born over. By the 1830s the object of romantic love had become effectively a challenge to God as the individual's main symbol of purpose. The meaning of life was focused on the love object and away from God and Christ. For right or wrong, romantic love itself became a kind of substitute for religion. Sex as the expression of romantic love became virtually a sacrament. So the act of sex gained importance beyond anything it had had before. Such a love was still pure: one adviser defined it as "Love in its truest, highest form." This was a "strong, unselfish affection." Yet it was "blended with desire—an honorable desire implanted by nature in the breast of men and women." As the historian Karen Lystra has observed, "Sex could be sacred and sexuality might be spiritual if affection were blended with desire." And although the procreative role of sexuality remained at the forefront, especially in an era of only primitive birth control, sex became more respectable as a means of recreation as long as the couple were in love. The minister Robert Burdette, for example, gave no suggestion that he felt his premarital intercourse with Clara, a respectable clubwoman, in any way violated her purity. As he explained in a letter to his fiancée, "your love ... so pure ... womanly in its ardent passion." Sexual expression enhanced romantic love.

For purity meant passion too. More than anything else, Victorian America was the era "when passion reigned." A number of letters have survived that confirm that purity did not mean repression but rather a passion that was refined, spiritual, and controlled. One young man declared that "my whole emotional being seemed merged in yours, robbed of you I should be poor indeed." Robert Burdette wrote of the intensity of his love for his girlfriend: "And when I have reasoned it all out and set bounds for your love that it may not pass, lo, a letter from Clara, and in one sweet, ardent, pure edenic page, her love overrides my boundaries as the sea sweeps over rocks and sands alike, crushes my barriers into dust out of which they were builded, over whelms me with its beauty, bewilders me with its sweetness, charms me with its purity and loses me in its shoreless immensity."

Victorian letters, because they were understood as part of the private sphere, often lacked the reticence of the public sphere. Lester Frank Ward wrote to his fiancée: "We lay with our faces together. I unfastened my shirt and put (her) tender little hands on my bare breast, and . . . she gave me her heart and her body, asking nothing more in exchange than my own." Women, too, might be just as honest. One woman wrote to her husband: "How are you this hot day? I am most roasted and my chemise sticks to me and the sweat runs down my legs and I suppose I smell very sweet, don't you wish you could be around just now?" This was mild, of course, compared with contemporary underworld standards or indeed with standards today. Still, the same woman referred in another letter to her lover's "old long Tom." Victorians understood how greater eroticism could be achieved in subtlety: "I could not help saying a few words . . . would that I could kiss you all over—and then eat you up." Victorians adopted a refined style that indicated they were playing within the rules: "If I don't behave with great impropriety then it will be for better reasons than I can now foresee. I'll just squeeze her and hug her, and kiss her forehead and eyes . . . and I'll take liberties with her back hair and pull out her hairpins, and tousle and tumble her up generally. . . . Won't that be nice, old Loveliness?" The Victorian stress on purity and romantic love meant that passion and desire held sway if kept within the rules of the culture of character. Victorian America was therefore a kind of heyday for heterosexual relations, a time when it was truly great to be straight.

While separate spheres applied in the public world, Victorian morality incorporated a rich world of intimacy for men among men and for women among women. The historian Carol Smith Rosenberg, in a famous essay written in the 1970s, first identified a "female world of love and ritual" from the late eighteenth to the mid-nineteenth century. Victorian women regularly formed intense emotional relationships with each other. Women's friendships helped communities jell and ensured social continuity. Elaborate networks of mothers, daughters, cousins, aunts, and assorted kin kept women going through good times and bad. At every major life event—baptisms, weddings, funerals—the women's network appeared. Such bonds as existed among women were not just emotional but also physical. One teenager wrote that "[she] laid with my dear Rebecca and a glorious good talk we had until about four [a.m.]. O how hard I do LOVE her." As another wrote to her cousin after her separation, "What would I not give just now for an hour's sweet conversation with you." Although such women's friendships could be found in any century, they gained a peculiar intensity in the nineteenth century when separate spheres between the genders was the norm. As one woman recorded in her diary in 1834: "I do not believe that men can ever feel so pure an enthusiasm for women as we can feel for one another." Above all, however, it was quite possible for women to form sexual lesbian relationships. Turn-of-the-century "Boston marriages" between women who lived their lives together could easily be assimilated into the norm of strong female friendships.

In turn, men formed their own world of intimacy and romantic friendship. Such was the language that men used with each other that it is impossible to distinguish friendships that were physical and erotic from those that were not. One young man wrote of another that "O yes John has an affectionate heart, a noble heart." Another wrote of his friend, "It is not friendship that I feel for him, or it is friendship of the strongest kind, it is a heart-felt, a manly, a pure, deep, and fervent love." Others addressed one another as "Lovely Boy" or "Dearly Beloved" or ended letters with "Accept all the tenderness I have." They reminisced that "the hour is arrived when you and I . . . used to pile up our books and converse with a fondness I always approve." Victorian relationships between men could be close.

Some such relationships therefore might have been sexual. The lover of young James H. Hammond, pillar of the Old South, wrote to him of his "poking and punching a writhing Bedfellow with your long fleshen pole—the exquisite touches of which I have often had the honor of feeling." Cross-generational relationships that were consummated and homoerotic were quite common too. An older man might see his young friend through college or else help him into his career before he married. Most men who felt their strongest feelings for other men married and perhaps continued to have affairs with their own gender. Other relationships, while intense and ardent, were not sexual but rather a support for a young man as he searched for the right woman to marry. According to a historian of manhood, E. Antony Rotundo, "they exchanged advice, they rhapsodized about feminine beauty, they cursed feminine wiles, and they consoled one another when romantic hopes were dashed." Yet the language they used with each other was so intense and emotional that real homoerotic relationships could have existed in this context without being identified as such. In Victorian America it was quite possible for a man to be in a sexual relationship with a man and for a woman to be in a sexual relationship with a woman but still to maintain respectability concealed behind the rhetoric of separate spheres and passionate romantic friendship.

But in the public sphere, Victorian sexual boundaries were very clear. Victorians insisted that men and women of character respect each other and obey the rules of propriety. They upheld a single standard of monogamy for both men and women, bolstered by the institution of marriage. Promiscuity was not respectable, nor were esoteric sexual practices. Sex before marriage was often tolerated in private among the engaged but not openly encouraged. While divorce laws were gradually relaxed over the Victorian period, divorce was still frowned on. Aware of the precariousness of the social structure they had created as they grew even further away from ancient Christian sanctions, Victorians stressed the importance of the family. This came at the cost of severe curtailment of women's freedom in the public world. But men too felt themselves burdened by the breadwinner's role.

Yet Victorianism worked. Rates of divorce and illegitimacy stayed low. And the family as a "haven in a heartless world" gave men and women the support necessary to build America in the nineteenth century. Victorian sexuality was, then, both an economic and a democratic triumph. And at the same time sex managed to be fun. Americans today may look back with nostalgia at the Victorians, for their system managed to create a healthy balance between sexual repression and sexual liberation.

But this success came at a price. The lofty, refined, spiritual middle-class virtues that helped to refine courtship and marriage for Victorians and became the essence of respectability were in marked contrast to the behavior of the "other Victorians" of the underworld that permeated America's teeming cities. Here was found not Victorian morality but immorality. Here played the "Fifth Avenue Parvenu, the preening Broadway dandy, the fancy gambler, the grasping Chatham Street

Jewish pawnbroker, the alluring prostitute, the streetwise newsboy." This lively and colorful society became the center-piece of a vast voyeuristic literature. A typical work of the genre was George G. Foster's *New York by Gaslight* (1850), which "promised to penetrate beneath the thick veil of night and lay bare the fearful mysteries of darkness in the great metropolis . . . the festivities of prostitution, the orgies of pau-perism, the haunts of theft and murder, the scenes of drunk-enness and beastly debauch and all the sad realities that go to make up the lower stratum—the underground story—of life in New York." Here was the antithesis of respectability, a world where men of both the middle and working classes in-dulged their vices—gambling, drugs, drinking, and sex with prostitutes. Victorians believed in the concept of male sexual necessity, that it was required of a society to provide prosti-tutes as a safety valve for men's primitive urges. If men could seek relief with prostitutes, they would be better able to culti-vate refined eroticism with middle-class women. Young men, unlikely to marry until their late twenties, provided the bulk of the brothels' customers. Everywhere prostitutes were given free admission to city theatres' uppermost galleries. After the Civil War, brothels proliferated at the edge of business districts and installed red lights outside; hence the phrase "red-light district," where such establishments received tacit acceptance from city government. Historians have surmised that half of American men in these years visited prostitutes at some stage in their lives. Victorian culture expected refine-ment and character from women, but it permitted men the freedom to indulge their primitive urges in secret. Respectable young men had no qualms about consorting not just with prostitutes but with other "lowlife" in the demimonde.

Nor was this underworld hidden away. Prostitutes dressed like ladies; they further confused and blurred the clear moral distinctions of the middle class: "They dress in great elegance, and quite as decorously as females generally do at balls, parties, or at concerts. Meet them in the streets, or at picture galleries, or at a fashion soiree, and there is nothing about them to attract attention. No person who knows them or their character can in any way recognize them in public." Hence it was possible for a respectable businessman or minister to be lured into a house of prostitution. And it was even possible for a "handsome and fashionably dressed street lounger" to seduce a respectable wife and then threaten to blackmail her husband. For this Victorian underworld acted not merely as a safety valve for male indulgences but as a counterculture that in its practice of loose living, deception, and promiscuity challenged the sobriety of the middle class. Worse, here lay the roots of a revolt against Victorian sexual morality: for this underworld was the absolute antithesis of the high standards of the public middle-class world of heterosexual courtship. And, though it played a key role in the Victorian system, it always threatened to subvert it.

There were other challenges. In the middle-class world of respectability, homosexual behavior could comfortably blend in as part of romantic friendship. There were no homosexual persons. But in the underworld of nineteenth-century America, a different and stereotypical homosexual identity was developing. Most of the evidence of this comes from sensational and voyeuristic tracts about the underworld. One described homosexuals as "beasts in human shape"; another referred to New York's "brutal sodomites and beasts who followed that unhallowed practice." Homosexual males not only indulged in corrupting sexual behavior but also behaved like women with their "weak" and "passive" roles. In Chicago at the turn of the century, homosexuals identified one another by their red ties. In the 1890 publication *The Vices of the Big City,* a homosexual bar was described as "the most disgusting place. The place is filled with from one hundred to three hundred people, most of whom are males, but are unworthy of the name of men. They are effeminate, degraded, and addicted to vices which are inhuman and unnatural." These early examples of homophobia undoubtedly helped establish in Americans' minds the existence of a particular and peculiar type of person defined by his sexuality. And this sense was solidified by the resistance of members of the subculture. The author of *A Cop Remembers* (1899) recalled how homosexuals in her district "caused [me] plenty of trouble." She went on: "Don't think for one moment that some of those fags can't put up a battle. I certainly miscalculated on some of them and one, especially, gave me more than I handed him. Just listen to this. Two of them came in one day and ordered milk punches with eggs. The bartender yelled, 'Nothing doing, get out of here!' When they got to the door, one of them turned and said acidly, 'We may be fags but we're no common bartenders anyway.' A barrage of lumps of ice was the answer from the bar." The members of this homosexual world dabbled in alternative gender roles and thus comprised a further counterculture that challenged Victorian morality from within.

Pornographers were a third counterculture. In the 1850s investigator William Sanger reported that in New York "boys and young men may be found loitering at all hours around hotels, steamboat docks, railroad depots, and other public places, ostensibly selling newspapers or pamphlets, but secretly offering vile, lecherous publications to those who are likely to be customers." Obscenity was a huge business in the nineteenth century. French picture postcards were common. So were condoms, dildos, rubber penises, and sexually explicit books. Posters were available in the larger cities. *Aristotle's Masterpiece,* with its detailed explication of the mechanics of sexual intercourse, between 1800 and 1831 went through sixteen editions. More openly pornographic was the hugely popular *Fanny Hill: Or the Memoirs of a Woman of Pleasure* by the

English author John Cleland. Such work upset the lofty, spiritual, romantic idealism of Victorian America.

A fourth counterculture was the "free love network" that existed even in the years before the Civil War. In 1856 the phrenologist James H. Cook wondered if "Legal Marriage [was] a far greater curse than African slavery?" "Yes, by far," he concluded. The free lovers took their lead from the French socialist thinker Charles Fourier, who believed that human passions, if permitted without rein, would produce social harmony. Free lovers insisted on "unconditional freedom for love." Fourier described how "they are perfectly willing that the heart shall decide for itself whether it will have one or more objects. . . . They believe . . . that variety in love is not only natural, but in the highest degree promotive of purity, happiness, and development." And free lovers went beyond this to advocate the abolition of marriage. Francis Barry, an Ohio abolitionist, wrote: "I am aware that you and others advocate a system that you call marriage, in which love is an essential feature. . . . The term 'marriage' has, by common consent, been applied to a system of which love forms no necessary part."

Although confined to the margins, buried in the dominant mores that for the time being withstood all such challenges, the Victorian underworld represented the worst nightmares of the "best people" in nineteenth-century America. If the dominant morality represented Americans' highest aspirations, the demimonde illustrated their lowest. The great success of Victorian culture was its ability to keep a lid on the underworld. This ensured social cohesion in a young and dynamic society. By contrast, the twentieth century saw the breakdown of the Victorian cultural system and the rise of a commercially led morality with its origin in the underworld. This revolt against Victorian sexual morality has steadily gained ground in American society over the course of the last century. But it has also provoked a powerful defense of traditional morality all along the way. This revolt against Victorian sexual morality and the battle to preserve it are the subject of the pages that follow.

For after 1870 the stresses in Victorian morality became more acute. The precarious consensus began to be challenged both from within and without. As the ordeal of the Civil War gave way to the twin traumas of Reconstruction and industrialization, middle-class stability could no longer be assumed. Still, early challenges to Victorianism were aimed at making its rigors tougher by establishing a single standard for both genders. The so-called social purity movement fought against efforts by doctors and public health authorities to enforce state-regulated prostitution in America's cities. A broad-based movement of clergy, former abolitionists, and women's suffragists successfully defeated a number of such bills in New York, Chicago, San Francisco, and Philadelphia. They then turned their attention to the abolition of prostitution itself through a nationally distributed journal, the *Philanthropist.*

The Women's Christian Temperance Union, founded in 1874, joined in the social purity crusade. Originally formed to encourage temperance as a means of strengthening the family, after 1879, under the leadership of Frances Willard, the WCTU began a much wider program of reform. From 1885 the movement set up a social purity department to establish a single standard of morality. This entailed, for example, protective work with young girls, including the formation of travelers' aid societies, the opening of boarding homes, and the establishment of social clubs.

Yet the WCTU also saw the reform of male sexuality as a major goal. Mothers were told to inform their sons "that their virginity is as *priceless* as their sisters'." In 1885 a group of

Episcopal ministers started the White Cross society to encourage purity among men. This organization, pushed strongly by the WCTU, soon established branches across the country.

At first advocates of social purity tried to achieve their aims through the force of moral suasion. But after 1885 they began to campaign enthusiastically for a sexual age of consent. In that year, in Britain, the Criminal Law Amendment Act had established a (heterosexual) age of consent as the age of sixteen. Hearing of this, American purity advocates found to their horror that in many American states the age was as low as ten. This discovery immediately regalvanized the social purity movement and stirred the WCTU into action because it gave both groups a clear and tangible goal: the raising of the age of consent.

On the face of it, the loose alliance of both women and male reformers represented an enhancement of Victorian mores. They supported the family and the high standards of the middle class. But in fact, by beginning the assault on the double standard, they helped undermine Victorianism. Victorians insisted not only on chastity for both genders but tolerated male sexual license. The purity advocates would have none of this: the male seducer of an underage girl, for example, should be punished as a "fiend," a "devil," a "wild beast," or, worse, a "moral monstrosity," they argued.

As social purity began to gain ground, other challenges to Victorian morality appeared. In 1872 a Connecticut dry-goods salesman, Anthony Comstock, set up the New York Society for the Suppression of Vice to enforce anti-obscenity laws. In 1873 Congress passed a law banning the "circulation of obscene literature and articles made of rubber for immoral use." During the 1880s and 1890s Comstock, in his guise as a U.S. postal inspector, organized the arrest of hundreds of people. He vigorously pursued his goal, but by naming the obscenity again and again with almost voyeuristic relish, he contributed to the weakening of the conspiracy of silence.

Public reticence about sexuality now came under fierce attack from a renewed and far more visible free-love movement. In the 1870s Victoria Claflin Woodhull led the most spirited assault on Victorianism yet. She fiercely attacked marriage as a barrier to love: marriage permitted sex outside of love for young people and checked loving sex between those who were not married to each other. But Woodhull's major contribution was her public declaration that the respected minister Henry Ward Beecher was having an affair with a married parishioner, Elizabeth Tilton. Woodhull fell afoul of an outraged Anthony Comstock when she gave out details in her journal *Woodhull and Claflin's Weekly*, aiming to expose middle-class hypocrisy.

Ironically, both Comstock's efforts and Woodhull's follies gave a boost to free love. Ezra and Angela Heywood used their journal *The Word* to encourage blunt discussion of sex: "Such graceful terms as hearing, smelling, seeing, tasting, fucking, throbbing, kissing and kin words, are telephone expressions, lighthouses of intercourse," they wrote. Comstock went after Ezra Heywood too, having him sent to prison for three years of hard labor. But other free lovers thrived. Moses Harmon in Kansas published *Lucifer, the Light Bearer,* which contained material on oral sex. Comstock condemned it, then he went after Harmon for publishing a letter discussing marital rape. Harmon was imprisoned briefly as a result of this prosecution.

The Heywood and Harmon trials adopted the so-called Hicklin test of obscenity (based on the 1868 English case of *Regina v. Hicklin*). This defined obscenity as "whether the tendency of the matter charged as obscenity is to deprave and corrupt the morals of those whose minds are open to such

influences, and into whose hands a publication of this sort
may fall." This was to be the litmus test against which later
liberalization defined itself. Although Comstock's intimidat-
ing tactics made him the curse of sexual liberals and libertari-
ans until his death in 1915, free love continued to attract
followers. Despite the clear challenge to Victorianism that it
posed, free love was still quite mainstream in its insistence that
"true love" could result in children who were both morally
and biologically superior: late nineteenth-century middle-class
Americans, proud of their Anglo-Saxon roots, were peculiarly
susceptible to such appeals.

A far greater challenge to the Victorian consensus in the
long term was the Irish playwright and aesthete Oscar Wilde,
whose visit to the United States in 1882 mobilized the anti-
Victorian forces as nothing had before. The visit, in which
Wilde promoted Gilbert and Sullivan's operetta *Patience* for
the D'Oyly Carte Company, was a sensation. Wilde found an
America in the throes of industrialization that welcomed a
new feminized style of masculinity and was beginning to see
same-sex intimacy in less sentimental and more erotic terms.
The idea of the invert or male homosexual as a persona was
beginning in the 1880s to enter common discourse. Wilde was
understood as part of a homosexual subculture that Americans were dimly aware of, but that Wilde now publicized with
relish and flamboyance. The *Brooklyn Eagle* noted that "the
pallid and lank young man, Mr. Oscar Wilde . . . will find in
the great metropolis a school of gilded youths eager to embrace his peculiar tenets." The *Washington Post* observed the
"gilded youths" with Wilde as "young men painting their
faces . . . with unmistakable rouge upon their cheeks." Fasci-
nation continued with reports of the meeting between Wilde
and Walt Whitman on January 18, 1882. The *Newark Daily
Advertiser* interviewed Whitman, who reported on their intimacy: "'I like that so much,' Wilde answered, 'laying his hand

on my knee.'" An account of Wilde's visit to the New York Stock Exchange also appeared homoerotic. The *Washington Post* noted Wilde's "form suggestive of corsets ... flowing tresses ... fresh from the oil jar, and rainbow stockings tucked into knee breeches." The paper went on to report that "about one thousand messenger boys crowded close around the aesthete" in an effort to get "Oscar on the 'floor'"; but they were "sadly disappointed" when Wilde fled out the back way. The *National Police Gazette* showed Wilde leading "newsboys and bootblacks." Wilde's connections to the demimonde were thus clearly visible.

A vogue for impersonation of Wilde now spread across the country. In Denver, journalists dressed up as Wilde; in Milwaukee, stock exchange dandies did so. A St. Louis grocer even proclaimed himself actually to be Wilde by dressing with flamboyance. Senator David Davis of Illinois "adopted" a newsboy without creating a scandal. Most Americans treated the visit with good humor. Even conservative journals such as *Harper's New Monthly Magazine* and the *Washington Post* reported on Wilde favorably.

Yet the defenders of Victorian morality could not fail to notice Wilde. Thomas Wentworth Higginson, in an article in the *Woman's Journal*—"Unmanly Manhood"—in February 1882, railed at both Wilde and the poet Whitman. He attacked Wilde for writing poems that "carry nudity." And these, he declared contemptuously, were "called 'manly poetry.'" Wilde responded by calling Higginson a "scribbling anonymuncule in grand old Massachusetts who scrawls and screams so glibly about what he cannot understand." Others criticized Wilde's aesthetic philosophy. Wilde elevated the ordinary American workingman into a sexually desirable art object. When he wrote of silver miners as "the most graceful things" who "might have been transformed into marble or bronze and become noble in art forever," he offended sensibilities. Comments like this provoked ridicule in some quarters: "Oscar Wilde says that every handicraftsman is graceful and beautiful when at work. This is sweet consolation to the boilermaker who crawls inside and stays to rivet bolts." Others understood the challenge to traditional sex roles that Wilde posed: "Mr. Wilde is an emasculator of ideas. His example would turn our young men into drawling asses and our maidens into puling idiots."

Wilde touched nerves in late Victorian America. But there was much else to the fast-developing challenge to Victorian morality. By the 1890s changes in feminine ideals helped to create the celebrated "New Woman" and the start of a revolution in women's identity. The natural curves of Richard Harding Davis's Gibson Girl drawings were typical of this New Woman. She was no longer meek and mild but enjoyed sports, dancing, and cycling. How long before she rejected purity? Other models of the New Woman seemed to suggest that the rejection would occur sooner rather than later. At Chicago's World's Columbian Exposition in 1893, the risqué Hootchie Cootchie Girls shocked. Male novelists began to present more daring images of womanhood. Theodore Dreiser's *Sister Carrie*, banned when it appeared in 1900, depicted its feisty heroine's rise to riches on the backs of men who themselves ended up in dissolute poverty. Stephen Crane's *Maggie: A Girl of the Streets* (1896) was a sympathetic portrayal of a prostitute. All this taboo-breaking by both men and women contributed to the development of an "American nervousness," a profound sense that older meanings and certainties were no longer relevant in an industrializing, urban society.

Changes in women's roles were rivaled in the late nineteenth century by a dramatic change in male life. According to one demographer, of men born in the decade 1865 to 1874, 37.3 percent remained single in the 1890s. This was an all-time high. Also, the average age of marriage for males in the year

1890 was 26.1 years, also unprecedentedly high. Bachelors congregated disproportionately in the major cities; in every city, with the exception of Denver and Baltimore, the number of bachelors was higher than the national average. And bachelors were disproportionately from the native-born population and not from the burgeoning immigrant population—that is, they came from those groups whose parents had espoused Victorian morality.

This trend had enormous implications. The Victorian system of morality had aimed to control male sexuality as much as to confine women. But with the appearance of a large bachelor subculture in the cities, such control no longer became tenable. Young men congregated in urban areas, crowding into bachelor apartments. The journalist Will Irwin recalled living "five in a room with two double beds and a single one. Here a strong social world developed around saloons, gyms, the YMCA, pool halls and barber shops." *Forum* magazine noted that "men's matrimonial discouragements and bachelor compensations are many." With a shrewd eye for the main chance, an entrepreneurial editor, Richard K. Fox, took over the *National Police Gazette* and turned it into what one recent historian has called "a combination of *Playboy, National Inquirer,* and *Sports Illustrated.*" It became the bachelor's bible. A late-1880s issue contained an editorial, stage gossip, portraits of female stage performers, a major tale of crime, sports columns, and ads for venereal disease cures. By the 1890s, photographs of coquettish young women increased: more and more crime stories appeared showing pictures of females wearing only lingerie.

Along with a surplus of men, the urban environment also contained a growing number of single women. From the 1890s, more and more young women began to take jobs as department store assistants and secretaries. With expendable income, young men and women began to take advantage of the growth of leisure: dance halls and amusement parks sprang up to meet the demand. By the 1890s an early form of a new heterosocial culture had appeared in America's cities. Here young men and women gained the freedom to enjoy themselves as never before. As the sociologist Ernest Burgess remarked, "In towns and cities marriage tended to be delayed, the period of courtship and engagement extended. With the growing economic independence of youth, their social life became an end in itself." This stress on leisure and pleasure contrasted directly with middle-class Victorian values. And businessmen recognized that youth was now ripe for picking. The revolt against Victorian sexual morality had clearly begun. Yet as the new century dawned, the emerging Progressive movement ensured that supporters of Victorian values could fight back with renewed vigor.

2

Bohemia, the War, and Birth Control, 1910–1920

IN 1913 *St. Louis Mirror* editor William Marion Reedy declared that it was "Sex O'Clock in America." In the *Atlantic Monthly* of March 1914 the essayist Agnes Repplier announced "the repeal of reticence." These two writers did not try to conceal their concern with the rush of discussion of the subject of sex. But others welcomed the new openness. The bohemian novelist Sherwood Anderson commented approvingly of the "healthy new frankness . . . in the talk between men and women, at least an admission that we are all at times tormented and harried by the same lusts." Another writer in the *Dial* of 1916 enthusiastically announced that Americans had been freed from "Victorianism" and pleaded, "Heaven defend us from a return to the prudery of the Victorian regime." Another author anxiously wondered whether "vice not often matched since the Protestant Reformation" could lead to a reversion to "Puritanism." If Virginia Woolf across the Atlantic had famously declared that "in 1910 the world changed," it seemed to American cultural critics in 1912 to 1913 that their world—the sure and certain world of Victorian morality—was crumbling.

In the years before World War I the "conspiracy of silence" around sexuality continued to unravel. Yet this was only the tip of an iceberg of social change. The possibility of marriage as personal fulfillment rather than the glue of social stability appeared in the new mass-circulation magazines, such as *Munsey's* and *Cosmopolitan*. Discussions of the growing divorce rate gave early evidence of a new twentieth-century morality, as divorce demanded a reconsideration of the Victorian image of the pure woman who was protected by the double standard. Women had rights too, and they used them to initiate divorce; they did not merely depend on men. By 1900 various writers were making public the radical proposition that women were not merely spiritual creatures but actually had sexual feelings. Many respectable Americans believed that the mores of the lower orders, injected with the massive influx of immigration from southern and eastern Europe, were gaining ground. Indeed, as nickelodeons, movie theatres, dance halls, and amusement complexes spread widely in America's teeming cities, it often seemed that older moral standards were being overwhelmed.

As the century entered its second decade, Americans thus turned to reform en masse in an effort to make sense of and order their changing society. The 1912 election saw a virtual consensus develop around the reform movement known as progressivism, as Woodrow Wilson's New Freedom triumphed over Theodore Roosevelt's New Nationalism. With the Progressives' mass support among the middle classes, the movement in many ways represented the culmination of Victorianism in American society: progressive Americans had an optimistic belief in the power of science and medicine to uplift and purify. The highest moral standards could be enforced by an elite of what they often called the "best people."

Yet the Progressives, like the social purity advocates before them, unintentionally weakened the older moral system they sought to preserve. The confrontation of venereal disease is a case in point. By the early twentieth century it was becoming increasingly clear that venereal diseases were a far greater problem than had previously been thought. Not only did the extent of infection among the population—about 10 percent—become appreciated, but the stealthy workings of tertiary syphilis and its link to many other diseases began to be understood. A group of doctors under the tutelage of Prince Morrow formed the American Social Hygiene Association in 1912 as an amalgam of other groups. The association aimed to teach the middle-class young about sex, believing that this was the best way to prevent disease. In doing so, it was among the first to break the taboo surrounding sex discussion. The ASHA also challenged the double standard in its organization that united long-established anti-vice crusaders and medical reformers in a vigorous attack on prostitution. Four major studies of prostitution appeared between 1911 and 1917 that gave focus to the association's efforts and helped weaken one of the key safety valves of Victorianism. A typical progressive organization in its stress on scientific uplift and elite-led efficiency, the ASHA undermined the pragmatic Victorian double standard by insisting on the ideal of a single standard of sexual morality for all.

At the same time another challenge of a very different kind came from New York's Greenwich Village radicals, who started to experiment with the ideas about sex of a number of European writers. Swedish writer Ellen Key, in her 1911 book *Love and Marriage*, justified the development of a new social system on the grounds that evolutionary progress demanded one. Because human nature had changed, so too should human morality. For Key, this meant that men and women should be free to experiment with their sexuality both before and after marriage. Love justified everything: "Love is the moral ground of sexual relations." This was nothing less than what Victorians had believed. Yet Key was different too. By naming the sex act and by suggesting that it was publicly acceptable outside of marriage, she favored frankness over Victorian hypocrisy. The youthful and idealistic Village bohemians read her work avidly.

Two British writers especially had an enormous effect on the Villagers. The first, Edward Carpenter, was a well-known figure in the cranky and wacky world of late nineteenth-century British socialism. Carpenter's sexual interests reflected the taboos that the British class system excited. He lived openly with a number of working-class men. Dubbed the "English Walt Whitman," Carpenter's major interest for Americans lay not in his pioneering homosexual style of life, which remained largely unspoken, but in his books such as *Love's Coming-of-Age* (1896), which, while their concealed aim was to encourage homosexual relations, redefined heterosexuality in the process. Carpenter, echoing Key, argued that "Sex is the allegory of love in the physical world." And while Key and Carpenter buried some of their ideas in semi-mystical language, with terms like "soul-passion" and "elective affinities," their message was clear to those eager to receive it: a new morality was necessary in order to free men and women to experience the heights of sexual love and passion. Like the nineteenth-century free lovers who in their time had tried to upset the Victorians, these writers likened the sex act to the creation of a utopian society. Their works appealed to idealistic young people because they suggested that improved relations and greater equality between men and women were a way toward a better society. Such folk would be moved by Carpenter's vivid description of the "sex act": "How intoxicating, indeed, how penetrating [sic], like a most precious wine— is that love which is the sexual transformed by a magic of the will into the emotional and spiritual?" Perhaps most alluringly, a couple so linked might roam sexually if they wanted to. Carpenter talked of a "marriage, so free, so spontaneous, that it would allow of wide excursions of the pair from each other."

A second influential British writer, Havelock Ellis, removed the ethereal language of Key and Carpenter and replaced it with a highly un-Victorian frankness and pragmatism. Ellis's *Studies in the Psychology of Sex* (1910–1928), a multivolume *tour de force,* made him into the foremost expert on the subject of sex in his day and perhaps of any day. Even more than Key and Carpenter, Ellis was a pioneer in a long tradition of intellectuals who sought to reform Victorian morality. Yet his work advised and recommended the whole gamut and range of erotic experience; he offered a sexual smorgasbord. He was the first widely known figure to stress the importance of the female orgasm and talk openly of "the various positions and techniques which were most likely to elicit it." Not only did Ellis extend and expand Carpenter's work on homosexuality, he also was the first medical authority to discuss sexual stimulation that might lead to orgasm—but not necessarily to procreation. He used his position as a medical doctor not only to divorce sexuality from reproduction but also to write of both oral and anal intercourse with all the authority of his rank. To Victorian Americans who had celebrated sex—but as refined, spiritual, and romantic—Ellis was deeply upsetting. To their children, however, he seemed to offer a brave new erotic world.

Ellis and friends found in Greenwich Village a receptive audience. In the decade up to World War I, these theorists' ideas took root among groups of youthful American radicals whose ability to express themselves was to give them great importance. The parlors of lower Manhattan welcomed after 1910 a formidable array of America's most talented youth. Fired in part by the tremendous burst of reformism that progressivism was bringing to the nation, they wanted to rebuild the world by dabbling in all the latest theories from Europe. They started *The Masses*, the irreverent socialist magazine which promised to build a new utopia in America. But as political nirvana remained elusive, they sought to change first their personal lives. Because they were rather spoiled, they were easily bored and gauged social progress according to the ebb and flow of their own personal happiness.

At the very center of the Village ferment was Mabel Dodge Luhan. Her celebrated salons acted as a catalyst to many of the impressionable, not to say gullible, but good-looking young people who arrived in New York after 1910 fired with vaguely socialist enthusiasms and with an earnest desire for love and romance. Here Havelock Ellis and Edward Carpenter were greeted as prophets for the future. Luhan's salon also introduced to many of the young the ideas of the founder of psychoanalysis, Sigmund Freud. Freud's tough-minded and rigorous insights that some sexual repression was necessary in order to maintain civilization, even at the cost of neurosis, may have seemed unlikely fodder to bohemians. But Luhan and her coterie found Freud's exploration of the unconscious appealing. They turned Freud on his head to interpret his complex and demanding work to mean that the solution to the neuroses that civilization could create was to have more and better sex—to avoid sexual repression at all costs.

This especially suited Luhan. The daughter of a wealthy Buffalo banker who, by dabbling in art and literature and conversation, sought in friendship and romance replacements for the sense of aimlessness she had always felt in an unloving family, Luhan found the most effective way of overcoming her boredom was by searching for ever more intense orgasmic experience. This need was perhaps made stronger because her first husband, Karl Evans, had been able to give her only a "single satisfactory experience," and that by accident. Her relationship with her second husband, Tony Luhan, offered apparently far superior sexual relations. As she herself described their first physical encounter, "I was by grace born in that flash as I should have been years, years ago; inducted in the new world." The historian Christopher Lasch observed, "She insisted . . . on the primacy of the particular sensations associated with sexual excitement. [She] may be regarded as a pioneer in the cult of the orgasm." For Luhan, sex was a vital part of her political plans: rejection of the staid and enclosing world of Buffalo from whence she came. A mature woman at the height of the ferment of radical ideas in the Village in the second decade of the new century, she inspired the idealistic young men and women who came to surround her. Her importance lies also in her introduction of the younger bohemians to the latest fads from Europe. Her craving for Key, Carpenter, Ellis, and Freud was as insatiable as her craving for young Village males. Luhan was a kind of catalyst for the new ideas about love.

Here, then, was the heart of the Greenwich Village bohemians' revolt against Victorian morality. These young people, privileged and articulate, had like Mabel Dodge Luhan fled to New York to find excitement they could not get in the great American heartland. They rebelled against their middle-class upbringing by becoming socialists and by advocating "modern love," which seemed to counter their parents' dullness and prudery. How they lived their personal lives was thus a key part of their politics. The new political and economic order that socialism would herald demanded a freer, more equal and open world of love, where the conspiracy of silence and the double standard were swept aside.

The bohemians therefore insisted on people's right to enjoy sex free from worries about reproduction. They demanded that women's sexual needs too should be given due care and attention. And, finally, they insisted on what the historian Kay Trimberger has awkwardly called "mutual sexual fulfillment with interpersonal intimacy" in a relationship of equals. In other words, like Key, Carpenter, and Ellis, they advocated sexual satisfaction, intimacy, and equality between men and women.

They also challenged monogamy by suggesting that a variety of affairs outside a main relationship was acceptable. Here lay the very hub of their difference from the Victorians. Victorian engagements and marriages were set in the context of families and communities. The privacy Victorians valued reflected age-old respect for the sacred mysteries of love. But the Greenwich Village bohemians now cast relations between men and women—or "relationships," as they called them—in the context of a larger political agenda that aimed radically to transform middle-class values. Relations between men and women were at the forefront of the bohemians' political and artistic battles; that is why they paid so much attention to sex. But the bohemians' relationships lost layers of depth: love itself became more temporary and lost much of its spiritual meaning. As the philosopher Hannah Arendt has noted, "Intimacy is a poor substitute for privacy." This the bohemians soon found out.

No wonder that, like their mentor Havelock Ellis, the bohemian men and women experienced sad, even tragic relationships. Because of their self-absorption, they have left us a mass of material on their affairs and romances. The men struggled to wipe out the effect of their upbringing; the women battled to live their lives freed from the Victorian protections that family and community had offered them. This was the sort of woman who appealed to *The Masses* editor Max Eastman, who wrote of his "unqualified liking for women with brains, character and independence." Yet ultimately Eastman preferred traditional women to the New Woman. His marriage to "New Woman" Ida Rauh was scarcely consummated before he found himself attracted to Ruth Pickering, who, at seventeen, was ten years younger than him. This attraction and others greatly upset his wife, and they later divorced. Eastman's next relationship was with the actress Florence Deshon: their arguments over her long-term affair with Charlie Chaplin, and Eastman's sporadic affairs, may eventually have contributed to her dramatic suicide. Eastman's miserable experience of the consequences of "modern love" eventually drove him back to traditional marriage in the same way that he became disillusioned with socialism and moved toward the Republican party.

Hutchins Hapgood, too, saw "open marriage" as a way of advancing human relations. As he wrote of his wife Neith Boyce in his autobiography *A Victorian in the Modern World* (1939): "To have her know other men intimately, was with me a genuine desire. I saw in this one of the conditions of greater social relations between her and me, of a richer material for conversation and for a common life together." But when Neith Boyce actually put this idea into practice, Hapgood became so angry that he became physically violent with her. Boyce struggled to adhere to Hapgood's insistence on affairs, but at heart she was a one-man woman. She wrote to Hapgood, "I assure you that I can never think of your physical passions for other women without pain—even though my reason doesn't find fault with you." The abandonment of Victorianism thus proved onerous and burdensome. It certainly didn't bode well for modern love.

Floyd Dell, assistant editor of *The Masses* and later a successful novelist, defined his ideal as a "woman that can be talked to and that can be kissed." Yet even he found "modern love" trying and difficult. His first marriage to an older Chicago feminist, Margery Curry, ended acrimoniously. The problem for him was that he found women who were intellectual and women who were "kissable." But never both!

In his autobiography, Dell described his dilemma: "My private life became a bewildered and inconsistent one. I fell in love, and very seriously; and my wife, however hurt, was kind and generous, and willing to end our marriage. It was I who refused to give up our marriage, and after desperate attempts to eat my cake and have it upon one theory or another, I gave up my love affairs to keep my marriage—only, against my will to fall in love with another girl, and give up that love, and then with a third, giving her up in turn." Felix Fay, in Dell's 1920 novel *Moon Calf,* discussed this conundrum: "'Why in the world should you not regard intellectual women as kissable?' 'I don't know,' confessed Felix. 'But the fact is, I like the others better. Perhaps my tastes are vulgar. I am more at home with them—I feel freer. But when I sit beside them in the theater, and hear them laugh at silly jokes, and feel their lack of appreciation of something a little subtle, I—well, I despise them.'" Faced with this dilemma, Dell retreated into a revised version of Victorianism. In 1919 he married B. Marie Gage who, while she had been a socialist, a suffragist, and a feminist, was happy to give it all up for Dell. By 1930, in his *Love in the Machine Age*, he had abandoned "modern love" altogether for what he called "adult love," that is, heterosexual monogamy. This was Victorian in most ways, but with a greater stress on equality between men and women.

The Greenwich Village bohemians, as leaders in the revolt against Victorian sexual morality, encouraged a liberation for both men and women from an imagined "myth of Victorian repression." In reality, however, they confined themselves to unsatisfactory "relationships," for old habits died hard.

The cultural fears and anxieties of the Progressives and bohemians reflected deep changes in the structures of American society. By the 1910s these were beginning to affect the mass of Americans. As the United States industrialized, the values of the older Victorian elites seemed more and more outmoded. Working for the corporations that sprang up, it was easy to become a faceless manager or bureaucrat or office worker. Bosses paid good salaries for work that was dull and unfulfilling. The spare cash gave the "new middle class" the chance to seek therapy in the rich and colorful world of mass leisure and pleasure that appeared in every city across the land. The late nineteenth-century pioneers of the "new amusements"— dance halls and movie theatres—had originally tried to attract the working class. Now they realized that the young of the new middle class too were willing to spend their money to have fun. This trend was to gain greater momentum in the 1920s, but it was well under way in the teens. And its importance for the revolt against Victorian sexual morality cannot be underestimated. The Progressives tried to preserve Victorian morality while inadvertently weakening it. But the proprietors of the new middle-class leisure world had few qualms. They drew on the Victorian underworld to build a new American sexual morality.

In this context of a culture in ferment, women's position changed most profoundly, both in the middle class and the working class. The critic and social commentator H. L. Mencken introduced the "flapper" in a 1915 article in the *Smart Set*. He described a woman who had not yet become a part of American folklore but who did sharply diverge from the imagined popular image of the Victorian Cult of True Womanhood as "pious, pure, domesticated, and submissive." By way of contrast, this flapper was worldly-wise and experienced: "Life, indeed, is almost empty of surprises, mysteries, horrors to this flapper of 1915." Most shocking was her difference from the female ideal of only the preceding generation, Charles Dana Gibson's celebrated Gibson Girl. The flapper, according to the historian Kenneth Yellis, "refused to recognize the traditional moral code of American Civilization, while the Gibson Girl had been guardian." The Gibson Girl had seemed "incapable of an immodest thought or deed," yet "the flapper strikes us as brazen and at least capable of sin."

The flapper challenged the Victorian role that had been assigned to women. But who was she? The flapper reflected the American woman's growing independence. More and more got jobs outside the home: in 1900, 23.5 percent of women had outside employment; by 1910, 28.1 percent. Approximately two-thirds of these women were single. Such women found they could afford to move away from their families and still have a little spare cash to enjoy the pleasures the city had to offer. The new world of heterosocial leisure and amusements offered a promise of excitement and fun. One historian has described the very un-Victorian "thrills" that were available in amusements parks, which by the 1910s were growing in number and attracting the middle classes: "Various amusements contrived to lift women's skirts and reveal their legs and underclothing, while numerous others provided opportunities for intimate physical contact." There was ample chance for "spooning" and "petting" on tunnel rides. Decorum disappeared. As a sign on one ride, known as the Cannon Coaster, wondered, "Will she throw her arms around your neck and yell? Well I guess, yes!" And she did.

Dance halls were places for young women to meet young men in order to find a "steady." "Spielers" were employed to interest the young girls while waiters saw it as part of their job to introduce young men and women. Usually they adopted the practice of "breaking." Girls would dance together in a line with men watching. The men would then seize an opportunity to separate the girls and couple off. The practice of "picking up" was adapted from street culture in order to find companionship for an evening. Men did not necessarily have to take the initiative. According to Hutchins Hapgood's investigation, there were plenty of "tough girls" who were ready to find men.

Most intriguing, though, was "treating," which the historian Kathy Peiss has identified among "charity girls." As a contemporary investigator explained, they "offer themselves to strangers, not for money, but for presents, attention and pleasure, and, most important, a yielding to sex desire." A waiter noted that "most of the girls are working girls, not prostitutes, they smoke cigarettes [sic], drink liqueurs and dance dis[orderly] dances, stay out late and stay with any man, that pick them up first." Here there was little decorum. There might be balconies or galleries above the dance floor where boys urged on by pressure from their peers could act rough. According to the historian David Nasaw, "Most of the sexual activity reported was consensual." While longer relationships might have developed, the environment encouraged those that were short, sharp, and sweet.

For women in Chicago, this practice was one of economic necessity: "If the girls are good and refuse invitations to go out, they simply have no pleasure." A department store saleswoman noted that "I might get invited out to supper and save twenty cents." Many women became cynical and called themselves "gold-diggers." One woman craftily made her dates pay her the wages she would have earned in her job that night, and then, having had a meal out of the man, would make some excuse and flee before giving him any sexual favors. As a Chicago man noted: "They draw on their sex as I would on my bank account to pay for the kind of clothes they want to wear, the kind of shows they want to see."

Such behavior was not as new as it might have seemed. American working-class women had always had more freedom than their middle-class counterparts. And many of these women were first- and second-generation immigrants who had no stake at all in American middle-class culture. Still, these women—feisty and vivacious—were openly breaking from Victorian expectations in that, first, they were proud and determined not to be prostitutes and, second, they were initiating changes that middle-class women were beginning to imitate.

Also in the vanguard of such changes were segregated African-American amusements and dance halls. Some of the larger of these welcomed whites and, according to David Nasaw, even "resegregated their establishments to make the whites feel more at home." There were also "black and tan" resorts where blacks and whites could socialize as they pleased, though only whites were allowed to dance to the black orchestra that played ragtime. Yet these dance halls, rare though they were, were on the cutting edge of what now clearly amounted to significant shifts in sexual mores.

By the second decade of the century there is much evidence that some middle-class women, as flappers, were copying the working class and African Americans and going to dances and new amusements in large numbers. The great pre–World War I dance craze permeated all classes. Vice organizations tried to ban the "Turkey Trot" and the "Grizzly Bear" until the great English dancers, Irene and Vernon Castle, were brought in to codify and formalize the rules for these dances so as to make them more respectable. Fears surrounded them because the music they used—ragtime—was a product of African-American culture with its perceived out-of-control sexuality. One hugely popular dance step was even called the "Nigger."

The middle- and upper-class flapper now asserted her sexuality in a way that would have upset Victorians. The practice of chaperoning and the elaborate set of rituals that had been involved in courtship declined. Writing in 1910, the novelist Margaret Deland noted a "Change in the Feminine Idea": "This young person ... with surprisingly bad manners—has gone to college, and when she graduates she is going to earn her own living. . . . She won't go to church, she has views upon marriage and the birth rate, and she utters them calmly, while her mother blushes with embarrassment." The etiquette adviser Dorothy Dix observed, horrified, that it was now "literally true that the average father does not know by name or sight, the young man who visits his daughter and who takes her out to places of amusement." Further, "nice girls, good girls, girls in good positions in society—frankly take the initiative in furthering an acquaintance with any man." Another novelist noted that "she is sure of one life only and that one she passionately desires. She wants to live that life to its fullest.... She wants adventure. She wants excitement and mystery. She wants to see, to know, to experience...." A coed diary written before World War I is particularly revealing of the extent of sexual practice among the writer's generation of college girls: "We were healthy animals and we were demanding our rights to spring's awakening.... I played square with the men. I always told them I was not out to pin them down to marriage, but that this intimacy was pleasant and I wanted it as much as they did. We indulged in sex talk, birth control.... We thought too much about it." Hard evidence of this exists too from sex research. According to Lewis Terman, nearly 90 percent of women born before 1890 were virgins at marriage, while of those born between 1890 and 1899, 74 percent were. Fifty-one percent of women born in the first decade of the century were virgins, and only 32 percent of those born after 1910. It is clear from these figures that middle-class Americans were already abandoning much of Victorian morality before World War I.

Progressive organizations would have none of this. Such agencies as the Committee of Fourteen and the Committee of Fifteen in New York and Chicago and, after 1914, the Bureau of Social Hygiene in New York tried to contain the new freewheeling morality. These progressive reformers worked out fresh methods of social analysis. They believed that empirical research would help them gather the information that they needed to lobby for city, state, and federal government reforms. Hence there emerged a bizarre figure: the dance hall investigator. These characters were hired primarily to find as much "dirt" as they could. But it proved to be difficult. A Mr. and Mrs. Hastings, investigating for the New York Committee of Fourteen in a September 1911 visit to the Terrace Garden, wrote: "We observed that a large majority of the girls came by themselves and the young men by themselves, each finding partners at the hall. Few introductions were seen; two girls danced together and two young men whose fancy they suit pick them out and dance with them." So far, so good. But the investigators were mainly interested in the small minority of boys and girls who left the dance halls together. It proved hard to discover salacious material on the halls, but, when they could, the investigators offered pornographic descriptions.

Chicago's Juvenile Protection Association investigators noted the dire affects of alcohol: "In one case the investigator saw a young girl held while four boys poured whisky from a flask down her throat, she protested half-laughingly all the time that she never had anything to drink before. A half hour later, her resistance gone, she was sitting on a boy's lap." They also observed elsewhere "a young boy, evidently new to the city, was seen looking for a [dancing] partner. He found one, a prostitute, who, after drinking with him all the evening, persuaded him to give up his job. At the end of a week she induced him to go with her to St. Louis to act as a cadet for a disorderly house." Such investigation, though it may seem to us voyeuristic, was well intentioned. Progressives engaged in a "search for order" in American society as the older cultural system broke down with the vast influx of immigration; the popularity of dance halls showed that the older system of courtship was disappearing and had not yet been replaced by the dating system that appeared in the 1920s.

Reformers were especially concerned about "the girl problem"—the rebellion against Victorian morality of working-class female teenagers. Robert Woods and Albert Kennedy, in their 1913 publication *Young Working Girls,* observed the "confusion of standards among adolescent girls, which is everywhere noted upon." Woods and Kennedy blamed the plight of teenage girls on their parents: "Training and knowledge which should be picked up in the home, have to be picked up in the street." Hence young girls rebelled by engaging in "showy dressing" and "loud talk" and got "into various forms of adventure with members of the other sex." The Committee of Fifteen concluded that young girls "experiment with immorality" because of boredom and "tedious and irksome labor." The Massachusetts Vice Commission complained that young girls "profess utter lack of respect for their parents and contempt for their home life. . . . Some of them are already willing and anxious to begin a life of professional immorality."

The Progressives, themselves very often women who had broken with gender conventions, could only preach female chastity as an ideal. They could see that the sexualization of young girls that was occurring in the urban centers was fertile ground for their induction into prostitution and other evils of the city they were trying to alleviate. The Progressives' discomfort with urban morals was nowhere more clearly displayed than in their campaign against "white slavery." Many Progressives believed that an international ring of pimps and procurers preyed on girls in American cities. A stream of books, films, and articles appeared between 1900 and 1914 with titles such as *The Great War on White Slavery, Fighting the Traffic in Young Girls, The Girl That Disappears,* and *House of Bondage.* In these tales, typically a native-born white girl who left the country for the city was tricked into a life of prostitution. No less than forty-four states enacted laws banning "compulsory prostitution" while in 1910 the government passed the "White Slavery" or Mann Act that prohibited the transporting of women across state lines for "immoral purposes."

Everywhere Progressives rallied to protect female virtue by regulating dance halls and new amusements through laws that limited alcohol sales, "tough dancing," and prostitution. The leader of the Committee on Amusements and Vacation Resources of Working Girls, Belle Lindner Israels, tried hard for protective laws in New York City while other women worked in Chicago and San Francisco. Progressives in New York founded the Girls' Protective League to encourage girls to spy on other girls at dance halls, new amusements, and motion picture theatres. They encouraged girls to behave morally; the *Survey* magazine reported that "Each girl is expected to become to some extent, her sister's keeper." Similar organizations sprouted in Cleveland, Detroit, Minneapolis, and New Haven.

Progressives battled boldly and fiercely against the commercialization of sex in the dance halls and new amusements, continuing the purity crusade begun by the social purity movement. But they had not counted on the emergence of the movies. Urban nickelodeons sprang up all over the United States in these years to cater to a largely working-class audience. By 1910 there were as many as twenty thousand in America's northern cities. An early film, *Lady on a Tightrope,* aimed at a peep-show audience; Thomas Edison's *The May Irwin Kiss* was said by Herbert S. Stone, a Chicago magazine editor, to be "no more than a lyric of the stockyard. Neither participant is physically attractive and the spectacle of their prolonged posturing on each other's lips is hard to bear. Magnified to gargantuan proportions and repeated three times

over it is absolutely disgusting. Such things call for police in-
terference." Still, the film found its defenders: "Kissing has
been a custom time out of mind," noted a New Orleans editorial. "That it should not be pronounced indecent is to open the
eyes of the world to a flaw in something they'd always held to
be without blame."

Soon the movies began to display even more overt eroticism. Between 1904 and 1906 the French studio Pathé issued a
series of films, *Naughty Subjects of a Picante Nature,* which
prompted a great deal of concern in the United States: "Most
[of these] films are evil. Their nature is without a single redeeming feature to warrant their existence. Not a single thing
connected with them has an influence for good. The proper
thing for the authorities to do is to suppress them at once,"
railed the *Chicago Tribune.* American-produced films such as
*How Bridget Served the Salad Undressed, College Boy's First
Love,* and *How They Do Things in the Bowery* stirred up no less
annoyance. Despite their claims to moralize and educate, they
really aimed to titillate. The YMCA declared in 1906 that
"Unless the law steps in and does for moving picture shows
what it has done for meat inspection, the nickelodeon will
continue to inject into our social order an element of degrad-
ing filth."

Such indignation at the content of the movies led to the first
demands for censorship. The New York Society for the Prevention of Cruelty to Children in 1908 declared that "Children support the picture shows at a cost to their little souls and
bodies and minds that no one can compute. The records of the
children's courts sadly prove this new form of entertainment
has gone far to blast the lives of girls and has driven many
boys to criminal careers." In the face of tirades such as these, in
December 1908 Mayor George B. McClellan announced that
"Each and every license for motion picture shows be revoked
and annulled."

By 1912 it was clear that these early efforts to censor the first flowering of the cinema had failed. A new generation of mainstream movie palaces was springing up to cater to the middle classes. This more sophisticated audience was no less susceptible to erotic motifs. Progressive social workers Louise de Koven Bowen and Jane Addams expressed fears of the movies' corruption of youth. The cinema, they argued, unleashed an "emotional force" which could serve as a "cancer in the very tissues of society and a disrupter of the securest social bonds." For as movie theatres spread into middle-class areas, they continued to titillate and excite. Silent films offered a fantasy of male and female perfection and a guide to courtship and romantic life that, while it often claimed to be Victorian and moral, represented in fact a parody of Victorianism that could seriously weaken the older moral system.

The actress Theda Bara briefly scandalized the new American middle class. Her image as an exotic "she-vamp," with her blatant sexuality, outraged respectable society: "I have never gazed into a face portraying such wickedness and evil . . . a face governed by the same muscular system as the serpent," noted one critic. Bara offended those in power: a film reformer insisted that he "would rather have my son stand at a bar and drink two glasses of beer than have him see that vamp woman. He may get over the effects of the beer in a week but he could not forget that woman until he was eighty years old." In this context, in March 1915 the Supreme Court opened the way for censorship of film by declaring that the movies were not protected by the free-speech provision of the First Amendment. They were "a business purely conditioned for profit" and were "capable of evil, the greater because of their attractiveness and manner of exhibition." As a result, various states now embarked on censorship campaigns. In response, the filmmaker D. W. Griffith produced a masterpiece, *Intolerance* (1916), which claimed to portray "the rise and fall

of free speech in America." Thus by the end of the Progressive
era the battle lines were clearly drawn: as commercial elites
challenged Victorian morality, Progressives tried to save it.
Yet, as with the social purity movement and the WCTU, by
naming the vice they too weakened a key tenet of the Victorian consensus: they contributed to the repeal of reticence.

The debate over birth control further exacerbated the revolt. Victorians, even women's rights activists, were not eager
to endorse the legalization of birth control. Yet, interestingly,
the birth rate was in decline throughout the nineteenth century, falling from an average of 7.04 children per woman in
1800 to an average of 3.56 per woman in 1900. There have
been many theories as to why this was so: the historian Daniel
Scott Smith has suggested that the decline was due to women's
increasing power to refuse intercourse—what he termed "domestic feminism"—and not to the use of contraception because it was not yet seen as respectable and was linked in
people's minds with prostitution and sexual immorality. Anthony Comstock had even persuaded Congress to pass an act
to forbid the sale of contraceptives. Still, historians agree that
contraception must have played at least a role in the decline of
the birth rate.

By the early twentieth century many commentators noted a
new attitude toward family size: "The modern idea is decid-
edly against the large families which were once in fashion, the
general opinion being that quality and not quantity should be
the determining factor." This new attitude partly reflected the
fact that the public health revolution of the late nineteenth
century had ensured that more children were living to adulthood. It was no longer necessary to have so many children in
order to have a few survive. Other influences worked in the
same direction. The emerging new middle class of the time
wanted extra money to purchase the burgeoning number of
consumer goods. They also wanted money for leisure and, not

least, for toys and presents for their children. And the working class simply could not afford too many children.

Margaret Sanger, long regarded as the leading propagandizer of birth control, devoted her attention first to the working class. Working as a nurse on the Lower East Side of New York, Sanger had been horrified by the number of unwanted pregnancies. She believed a good deal of misery might be prevented if lower-class women—often, of course, in those days from European peasant backgrounds—could learn how to avoid pregnancy. She specifically aimed her journal, *The Woman Rebel,* at the working class and at immigrants. There were good medical reasons why lower-class women should have smaller families. Why shouldn't the working class be able to put into practice what the Victorian middle class had been doing for decades?

Sanger did not, however, confine her work to offering advice on birth control. Inspired perhaps by her affair with Havelock Ellis, she became one of the leading advocates of the importance of female sexual expression which, like the Greenwich Village bohemians with whom she mixed, she saw as a vital part of the road to a socialist utopia. According to the historian Leslie Fishbein, "She came to view birth control as a weapon in the class struggle." If workers could limit their numbers, this would reduce the pool of labor to be exploited. But because women's freedom would be a necessary part of the socialist utopia, coitus interruptus and the desensitizing condoms of those days were insufficient methods of birth control; women must be able to enjoy sex. Hence Sanger searched high and low for less inhibiting methods of birth control, such as the cervical pessary.

Another prominent figure in the birth-control movement was the anarchist Emma Goldman. Like Sanger, she too had been shocked by the suffering of working-class women on the Lower East Side. Goldman had been first (in 1915) to explain to the public how to use contraception. She and her lover had been arrested and sentenced to time in the workhouse and, in her lover's case, a crippling $1,000 fine. Yet this did not deter her from continuing to disseminate birth-control information.

By the 1920s Sanger had abandoned her earlier association with Goldman and anarchism and also with Greenwich Village socialism. But she continued to insist on making information about contraception available to women who needed it. So she produced a number of works, such as *Happiness in Marriage* (1926), that encouraged women, once they had birth control, to relax and enjoy sex. She moved further from her roots in the pain and suffering of the working class to an advocacy of all women's right to sexual expression and the right to control their own bodies: "It is none of a society's business what a woman shall do with her own body." Sanger thus pioneered what the historians John D'Emilio and Estelle Freedman have called "sexual liberalism," the idea that private matters are not the concern of society.

Sanger, an able self-publicizer, has perhaps received too much credit as the main propagandist of birth control. She was prepared to break the law if need be. But there were other approaches. Her main rival, Mary Ware Dennett, refused to break the law and was appalled by Sanger's tactics. The two camps clashed. Once when Dennett went to the police station to help gain Sanger's release, she was assaulted by an associate of Sanger: "This is *our* affair, we don't want you in it." Yet Dennett deserves much of the credit for the emergence of the birth-control movement. A pamphlet she wrote for her two sons entitled *The Sex Side of Life* was first published in a medical journal and then was printed for a wider public when it was banned from the mails in 1922 as obscene. Yet Dennett persisted in selling copies of it, and eventually in 1929 she was indicted for sending obscenities through the mails and fined $300. In a landmark decision in 1930, the Second Circuit

Court of Appeals overturned her conviction on the grounds that her pamphlet was educational. This opened the way for sex education material no longer to be regarded as illicit. Dennett's defense was significant. She argued that it was necessary to talk of sex not in terms of "love" or "lust" but to make it clear that "the climax of sex emotion is an unsurpassed joy, something which rightly belongs to every human being, a joy to be proudly and serenely experienced." The word "joy" had previously carried connotations of spiritual ecstasy and intensity; it was not deemed appropriate for descriptions of sexuality, where "love" or "lust" were thought to be more suitable. Her use of the word prefigures a title like *The Joy of Sex,* a 1970s best-seller. Dennett, for all her determination to stay within the law, was no less subversive of Victorian values than Sanger. She wanted the fun of sexuality to be emphasized so that women would not grow up repressed by "civilized morality." While Sanger understood a woman's right to control her own body as well as her right to sexual pleasure, Dennett looked ahead to the cult of the orgasm.

By 1917 the revolt against Victorian sexual morality was well under way. This works against the older views that World War I was the major turning away from the Victorians. Nevertheless the impact of World War I should not be underestimated. It was during the war that the Social Hygiene Association and the anti-prostitution movements became agencies of the government in a massive campaign to prevent the spread of venereal diseases among the troops. The government set up the Commission on Training Camp Activities (CTCA), made up of experienced social hygienists. The CTCA followed the axiom that sex education was the best way to prevent venereal diseases. Commission doctors assumed that the soldiers were ignorant about sex, so they made it their goal "to educate these boys in the vital subjects of reproduction, sex hygiene, venereal diseases, in the teaching of which their parents and home communities have been so woefully negligent." They believed that such education would persuade the troops to abstain. CTCA official H. E. Kleinschmidt summed up this optimism when he wrote, "Cynics and self-made philosophers have failed to convince us that the sex urge, which is admittedly a primitive instinct, can no more be stemmed than the tide of the sea."

This sounds remarkably Victorian. Continence for men was the very linchpin of the CTCA's beliefs. As one pamphlet put it bluntly, "Sex power is not lost by laying off." The idea of male sexual necessity was described as "a grand old dodge with whiskers on it. . . . When I hear a fellow pulling the old health yarn, I'm inclined to keep him away from my sisters." But there was a subtle though important new tone. One lecturer urged soldiers to "live strong and clean" but also to "save every drop of your strength and manhood for the supreme experience." In other words, sex—albeit procreative sex within marriage—should be fun. The idea was to fight for Uncle Sam in order to come home fit for good sex. Victorians would have never publicly expressed enthusiasm for sex in this way.

There was more. The lectures of the CTCA at times in their graphic detail actually became prurient: "Does any red-blooded man feel any doubt of his ability to preserve his manhood though tempted by the alluring seductions or voluptuous and beautiful women in the whirl and excitement of the gay metropolis, or the fascinations that may come to you from delicate and devoted attentions in the solitude of remote billets?" Who could not have resisted acting-out following such a lecture? How long could the Ohio farm boy remain innocent in such an environment? The contradiction showed the dilemma that the CTCA faced in having to follow official public values and yet reduce the incidence of venereal disease among the troops—which, as in the later medical crisis of AIDS, required talking about the sex act itself. Inevitably, innocence was lost. And this loss of innocence went beyond the war zone. Newspapers now printed words like "gonorrhea" and "syphilis" as they had never done before. The elderly matrons of Peoria and the Babbitts of Wichita could read all about it and have their prurience satisfied.

World War I was significant in other ways. As part of its determination to enforce a single standard of morality for both sexes because of its fears about venereal disease, the government directly attacked the double standard of morality by rounding up prostitutes. The CTCA claimed that it destroyed 110 red-light districts during the course of the war. One madam wrote that "Gals are scarce as hen's teeth; they won't work in a house, the government has them buffaloed." Smugly the CTCA reported that "it is a little difficult to realize that a year ago these places constituted the overshadowing menace to the health and efficiency of the forces of the United States."

Thus the American army, while still in the United States, could not, as armies have always done, attract hordes of prostitutes. But in fact "Charity Girls" and "patriotic prostitutes" did follow the soldiers around, further helping to alter the patterns of courtship. And the soldiers willingly went along. Taxis were reported taking couples to secluded sites. In the flurry of patriotism, the appeal of a man in uniform proved too much for some. One girl was reported as saying that she "felt she was doing her bit when she had been with eight soldiers in a night." This was noteworthy because many of these girls were from respectable middle-class homes. This upset the simple class-based Victorian dichotomy that working-class girls were bad while middle-class girls were good. The flappers had arrived.

Once the American Expeditionary Force arrived in France, the temptations became even more visible. Social hygienists tried very hard to continue the message of chastity, most effectively telling the boys of the consequences for their families back home and their girlfriends if they became diseased. Their campaign was extremely effective: venereal disease rates among U.S. troops were far lower than among their European allies. No doubt this also reflected the continued strength of Victorian morality. But the appeal of France did make an impact. It was bound to. The war, itself, perversely, held an erotic charge. The American soldier was well aware of the casualties his French and British counterparts had taken. He knew that his life expectancy on the Western Front was low. And so for many the lures and temptations of France proved too enticing. If life might be cut short, why not experience it? And many of the soldiers who survived brought back to the United States a taste for what France had taught them. Was it the advanced erotic techniques of the prostitutes? Or the imagination of French pornography? Either way, by the end of World War I the Progressives' attempt to preserve Victorianism and to rein in the considerable forces that challenged it were becoming unmanageable. By the 1920s the anti-Victorian forces gained the ascendancy, building on the advances of the prewar period.

3

Flappers and Philosophers: The 1920s

SINCE Frederick Lewis Allen's classic commentary on the decade, *Only Yesterday* (1931), the 1920s have enjoyed a special place in the imagination of Americans. Partly because of its contrast with the dourness and belt-tightening of the depression-ridden thirties, the period has become associated in the popular mind with unrestricted hedonism: flappers, the revolt of youth, dances like the Charleston, the syncopated rhythms of jazz. These things seem to characterize an era when people were merrier, when life was easier and simpler, an interregnum between the rigors of war and depression.

There is much truth in this view. In recent years, however, our understanding of the decade has become more sophisticated. We can now see it as a way station on the route from a nineteenth-century culture of production to a twentieth-century mass consumer culture.

What did this transformation entail? Most crucially it meant that Victorian virtues and values had a good deal less relevance in the twentieth century. Thrift, sobriety, self-sacrifice, delayed gratification, and control of sexuality seemed the right standards for young men and women setting up their businesses or expanding America's frontier. But now, as cities grew and industrialization proceeded apace, large corporations with offices in the skyscrapers that dotted cityscapes had no need for the qualities of capitalist entrepreneurs.

Rather, they required bureaucrats and salesmen. Such men—and, increasingly, women—lacked the independence of the self-made man. They got ahead by kowtowing to their boss, by demonstrating charm and personality as well as competence. Having "character" did not become irrelevant; qualities such as self-control and discipline could not disappear from any functioning society. But a competing set of values became ever more important. As mass-production techniques revolutionized the workplace and Americans moved away from a culture of scarcity to one of abundance, the challenge for corporations was to sell their goods. The advertising industry grew in volume as more leisure time led to increased consumption. Advertisers promised relief and excitement from boredom if you purchased their goods. And an army of experts—doctors, psychologists, marriage counselors—grew to calm the vague sense of dissatisfaction and discontent that Americans felt at dull, white-collar work.

These changes heralded a new sexual morality. The higher and steadier incomes gained from new middle-class jobs provided the wherewithal for fulfilling hedonistic wishes. Sexual pleasure was one of the main carrots that advertisers and experts, doctors and ministers offered Americans to cope with the lack of meaning that men felt at work and that women experienced at home. This trend, well under way in the Progressive era with the challenge to the conspiracy of silence, the movies, dance halls, birth-control advocacy, Greenwich Village bohemians, and New Women, came to fruition in the 1920s. The attack on Victorian morality gained renewed vitality as moviemakers, writers, authors of sex manuals, and advertisers stressed youth and "sex appeal" as twin pillars of a new moral agenda.

The movies continued to pace this new morality. Douglas Fairbanks, Sr., the first male movie star, was clean-cut, all-American, and gentlemanly, even wholesome. His films dramatized a classic battle between good and evil. Yet he very consciously rejected respectable Victorian morality. Athletic and energetic, he took pleasure in his physical, even primitive, self. He enjoyed showing off his perfect body and lounging in athletic clothes. Gone was the stuffy male image of the past as Fairbanks in the teens and early twenties came to be the premier role model for American men. In a series of hugely popular films and an array of success tracts, he preached redemption through physical activity, sport, fighting, and sex. One of his films went so far as to promise "a new kind of love-making." In *The Nut* (1921), a frustrated and bored New York office worker finds a mate in a sophisticated bohemian girl "who enjoys the high life."

In his life as much as in his films and tracts, Fairbanks redefined American social relations between the sexes through his marriage to Mary Pickford, one of the most successful female stars of all time. Pickford was "America's sweetheart," epitomizing the New Woman. In *Behind the Scenes* (1914) she played a girl from a small town who comes to the city in search of work. Bored in an office, she joins a cabaret troupe and soon finds a boyfriend who takes her to restaurants and nightclubs. They marry, but he returns with her to his family, where she must be a housewife. This work exhausts her. She flees again to Broadway where she becomes famous. This does not prevent her from being raped by a producer; then her husband returns, and they agree to patch up their marriage. In the style of the time, the film contains clear warnings about women's emancipation, yet it is notable for its honest portrayal of a more liberated and independent woman. The moral message is undercut by the alluring portrayal of immorality.

Fairbanks and Pickford's life together echoed their movie roles and came to symbolize aspects of the new morality. Their divorces from previous spouses were openly discussed. Pickford declared that her ex-husband had been a violent drunkard. When they honeymooned in Europe, the press hounded them as "America's golden couple." Fairbanks and Pickford's private life literally became public as they established their show home, Pickfair, in Hollywood. The press watched and examined every move of America's first bona fide movie stars. Magazines printed pictures of their Pickfair estate in all its intricacy and elaboration. Everyone assumed that the couple's joy would last like a fairy tale—forever. But after ten years this marriage, which was to be a blueprint for many other Hollywood marriages, ended in divorce and tears.

Fairbanks and Pickford typified the new freer roles for men and women and a new marital ideal promoted by the burgeoning motion picture industry, and they helped pioneer a cult of celebrity through which Hollywood was to challenge Victorian mores. Cecil B. DeMille's films represented another influential reshaping of sexual morality. The bathroom scene in his *Old Wives for New* (1918) was so daring that it almost led to the abandonment of the film. His *Male and Female* (1919), which contained brief scenes of nudity, has been called "more daring in its subject matter than any other picture Hollywood has produced." DeMille turned this film into a "lavish Babylonian fantasy" which featured a king throwing his mistress into a lion's cage. In *Manslaughter* (1922), DeMille grappled with the contemporary decline in moral standards. A young flapper, following a joyride that goes terribly wrong, is charged with manslaughter. The judge connects her fate to a collapse in sexual morality reminiscent of the Roman Empire. This is an excuse for an "educational" Roman orgy with scantily clad actors and actresses. As Betty Blythe described her leading role in *Queen of Sheba* (1921): "I wear twenty-eight costumes and, if I put them all on at once, I couldn't keep warm." DeMille's favorite subject was adultery, which he explored in a number of films such as *Why Change Your Wife?* (1920) and *Forbidden Fruit* (1921). In the tradition of the day, he warned the audience of adultery's dangers. DeMille specialized in making his films as titillating as possible behind the veneer of a moral lesson. His work showed a lingering tension between old and new values. Americans wanted excitement, but they also expected sin to be punished.

By the 1920s the youth and flapper film had become a Hollywood favorite. Such films handed out advice on how to be single, just as DeMille had advised married couples about their relationships. The most influential of these films was *Flaming Youth* (1923), starring Colleen Moore. At the time the film was regarded as extremely daring. Moore's character, Patricia Fentriss, insists throughout on protecting her virtue. Yet the portrayal of dissolute "flaming youth" concerned only with petting parties was shocking. Fentriss, for example, dances and preens with gay abandon. Youth, it seemed, was quite happy to dispense with ancient moral codes.

Clara Bow, the "it" girl, extended the flapper genre to its limits. Bow made a number of films in the late twenties in which she played working-class flappers. The question on everyone's lips, of course, was, What was "it"? The movies insisted that "it" was "that quality possessed by some which draws all others with its magnetic force. With 'it' you win all men if you are a woman." Bow's naturalness convinced the public that she, at least, had "it." As one recent critic has observed of her style: "A playful pout. An alert, mischievous glance or toss of the head. The way she kisses puppies and cuddles children or descends from cars, her tiny feet in perpetual jazz-baby motion. It's endearing, and her warmth and unselfconsciousness as an actress seems natural even today." The message to young American women at the time was that they too could have "it." Bow was helping to create a sexier image for women.

But what about men? For all his energy and dynamism, Fairbanks was a little too calculated—and a little too old—to be the epitome of youthful male sexuality for the 1920s. The movies had to look to Europe to find the great Latin lover Rudolph Valentino, who was perhaps more subversive of Victorian values than any movie star yet. A Hollywood columnist noted of him: "You've heard of various animals hypnotizing others by the slow rhythmic motion of their bodies, just so does Valentino charm all those who come under his influence by the wonderful perfection of his every movement." In *The Sheik* (1922) he ravished an Englishwoman in his role as an Arab sheik. This worked on American male fears that the exotic was somehow more virile and more sexual. That Valentino's sheik was exposed as an Englishman only added to the confusion: this was very un-Anglo-Saxon behavior. Valentino in fact posed a problem for American men. Should they emulate the exotic and the primitive in order to be more attractive to women? One twenty-two-year-old certainly thought so: "I studied his style. I realized that nature had done much less for me in the way of equipment than she had for the gorgeous Rodolpho, but I felt that he had a certain technique that it would behoove me to emulate." Above all, Valentino upset Victorian and Anglo-Saxon images of manhood because his message was to be like him and get the girl.

Commentators had no doubt of *The Sheik*'s impact. In a lecture on "What the Films Are Doing to Young America," the sociologist Edward Alsworth Ross wrote that "more of the young people who were town children sixteen years ago or less are sex-wise, sex-excited and sex-absorbed than of any generation of which we have knowledge. Thanks to their premature exposure to stimulating films, their sex instincts are stirred into life years sooner than used to be the case." Concurring, high school teachers in the Lynds' *Middletown* believed that the movies brought "early sophistication" to the young with films such as "*Alimony*—brilliant men, beautiful jazz babies, champagne baths, midnight revels, petting parties in the

purple dawn—*Married Flirts*—Husbands, Sinners in Silk—
Women who give." The local newspaper noted that "Sheiks
and their Shebas sat without a movement or a whisper
through the presentation. . . . It was a real exhibition of love-
making and the youths and maidens of Middletown who
thought that they knew something about the art found that
they still had a great deal to learn." One working-class mother
went so far as to claim that the movies helped her to bring up
her daughter: "I send my daughter because a girl has to learn
the ways of the world somehow and the movies are a good
safe way."

At the same time Hollywood was developing a growing
reputation for immorality. Its most celebrated instance involved Fatty Arbuckle and the actress Virginia Rappe, who
died during a wild party that Arbuckle held in San Francisco.
It was charged that Arbuckle's weight was responsible for her
death during a lurid sex scene. When the director William
Desmond Taylor was discovered dead, newspapers blamed a
life of sex and drugs. These torrid events fueled a revived
movement for federal censorship of the movies, led by
the Women's Christian Temperance Union, the Reverend
William H. Short's Motion Picture Research Council, and
Canon William Chase's Federal Motion Picture Council.

In response, Hollywood moguls formed the Motion Picture
Producers and Distributors of America and chose as their
spokesperson Will Hays, a former postmaster general. Hays
was a brilliant choice because of his solid Midwestern conservative persona and his genuine flare as a publicist. He was able
to deflect criticism of the movies for a while, but the "morals
clause" he demanded that moviemakers sign amounted to
very little, for he insisted on the principle of "self-regulation."
In 1926 Short and Chase led a delegation to Washington to demand that Congress regulate the movies. But for the time
being these demands went nowhere.

In the theatre, meanwhile, the spectacular career of Mae West challenged the respectable at every turn. West's roots lay firmly in the traditions of the New York demimonde, where in the teens she had become renowned as a burlesque performer who refused to compromise in the face of efforts by reformers to tone her down. As a keen performer of the Grizzly Bear and the Turkey Trot, West brought "lower-class indecency to the foreground." By the mid-1910s she had moved her act beyond the confines of the Bowery to Keith's national circuit of variety theatres. As her biographer Mary-beth Hamilton put it, "With her multiple lovers and saucy looks, West displayed sheer indifference to middle-class standards."

In the mid-1920s West took her act to the mainstream theatre in a series of sensational plays that forever changed what was permissible on the American stage. She took advantage of a genre of "sex plays," such as *The Shanghai Gesture* and *Lulu Belle*, that by 1925 had become popular on Broadway. But West's play *Sex* (1927) outdid them all. Critics who had previously been measured in their response to the "sex play" now could not contain their shock. One described the play as "not sex but lust—stark naked lust." No wonder, for *Sex* gave to Broadway the innuendo and raunch of lower-class burlesque. West's character Margy Lamont was an unashamed prostitute: "Sailor Dan from Kansas, Sailor Dan from Kansas—oh Sailor Dan from Kansas. Yeh Sailor Dan from Kansas, flat feet, asthma, check came back, o, baby, I'll make you a present of that bird, he's yours." The subject was obviously prostitution.

For her next play, *The Drag* (1927), West went even further. She introduced to a middle-class audience the homosexual underworld. She cast her players from visits to Greenwich Village gay bars, and the play itself was in large part the product of the camp humor and innuendo of the players:

CLEM: Why you big Swede. You'd take it through a funnel if anybody would give it to you.

WINNIE: Funnel? That's nothing. I take it through a
hose. Whoops!

The Drag introduced a complete compendium of the gay underworld. The character Clem chased a straight-looking taxi
driver whom he described as "rough trade." Here was obviously a heterosexual man who worked as a male prostitute. If
in *Sex* West had been a blatant prostitute, now she adopted the
persona, lifted from the gay underworld, of the drag queen.
Her style was that of a woman playing a man playing a
woman. Here was a compelling character, one who was to be
imitated again and again down to the present. No wonder that
West's recent biographer has observed that her plays were "the
theatrical equivalent of a slumming excursion" for the middle
class.

West's third play, *Diamond Lil* (1932), was even more subversive because, while it did not suffer the raw reputation of
her previous work, it gave her critical respect. Hence an even
broader middle-class audience was attracted to it. Yet West
continued here the persona she had perfected in *Sex* and *The
Drag*. She played the mistress of a New York nightclub owner
involved in "white slavery." This play contained some of
West's most famous lines: "I always liked a man in uniform
and that one suits you grand, why don't you drop in and see
me sometime?" and the immortal "You can be had," and
"Goodness, what beautiful diamonds."—"Goodness has nothing to do with it." With West, the innuendo of the street
reached Broadway.

In American literature there appeared a similar frankness.
Perhaps the publication of 1916 of Theodore Dreiser's long-
suppressed *Sister Carrie* was the first indication of change in
acceptable norms for the representation of women. When F.

Scott Fitzgerald, a graduate of Princeton, published *This Side of Paradise* in 1920 to much acclaim, it seemed to many that a veil had been lifted. People were genuinely shocked by one female character's revelation that she'd "kissed dozens of men. I suppose I'll kiss dozens more." Amory Blaine, the hero of the novel, said he "saw girls doing things that even in his memory would have been impossible: eating at Three O'Clock, after dance suppers in impossible cafés, talking of every side of life with an air half of earnestness, half of mockery, yet with a furtive excitement that Amory considered stood for a real moral let-down." As Fitzgerald himself noted, "None of the Victorian mothers had any idea of how casually their daughters were accustomed to be kissed." Fitzgerald's tales of aimless, dissolute youth shocked America until, by the mid-1920s, he moved on to other things.

Fitzgerald played a brief, secondary role in the revolt against Victorian morality. Other American writers in the 1920s developed the revolt much more convincingly. Many of the group were former Greenwich Village bohemians who, having experimented and dabbled with varieties of relationships, decided to write about their experiences. These men, by now largely in their thirties and forties, were obsessed with their youth and in a series of works examined male initiation into relationships with women. Ludwig Lewisohn, in *Stephen Escott,* wrote that he was "without admitting it to myself, sex-starved; more than that; nothing had fed the estimation of the budding man." These writers attacked marriage too. Floyd Dell criticized the institution, using cockney rhyming slang, as a "briary bush." His protagonist, Felix Fay, feared marriage as soul deadening: "No doubt the old man meant well, but it scared me. I saw myself settling down in that little town and buying a house for that girl to live in."

The hero of Harry Kemp's quasi-autobiographical *Tramp-*

ing on Life (1922) delivered "a long harangue against marriage" as he traveled around, working as a sailor, a boxer, moving from port to port. Chicago-based Ben Hecht, in *Erik Dorn* (1921), described a dance-hall contact he had made: "She's not a woman. . . . She's a lust. No brain. No heart. A stark unhuman piece of flesh with a shark's hunger inside it."

And these male writers unashamedly depicted violence against women. Kemp at one point charged his love, Opal: "I caught her violently into my arms. I would plead and whine no more. I would take her by force. She fought hardily against me." When she screamed, he could only declare, "I love you and I'll kill you—or myself—or both of us—you've got to become my sweetheart." In Sherwood Anderson's *Many Marriages* (1923), the hero Webster rapes his daughter because her mother has refused to have intercourse with him. As Anderson commented sourly: "There was a kind of cruelty in nature, and at the proper time that cruelty became part of one's manhood."

This "revolt from the Village"—to borrow the critic Frederick Hoffman's term—permanently altered the portrayal of the relations between the sexes in American literature. And its success emboldened others to go still further. James Branch Cabell's *Jurgen* (1919) was a "romance" set in medieval times that was, even by today's standards, soft pornography. Despite its setting in the dim and distant past, it caused a commotion. Anita Loos's *Gentlemen Prefer Blondes* (1926), the story of two kept women and their gentlemen friends, created a scandal upon its publication in 1927. Other works raised the ire of censors when efforts were made to convert them into films. Ernest Hemingway's *A Farewell to Arms* (1929) was attacked for its scenes of "illicit love" in its account of a hospital nurse who has a love affair with her patient. Moralists were up in arms that in *The Sun Also Rises* (1926) Hemingway often used the term "bitch." William Faulkner's 1929 work *Sanctuary* caused him to lose his position as a scout leader. Censors described it as a "morbid tale of rape, murder, sexual impotence, and perversion." This description was not far wrong. The heroine Temple Drake first becomes involved with a no-good boyfriend and later is raped by a ne'er-do-well named Popeye, who runs a brothel in New Orleans. But Temple actually enjoys the rape and starts a relationship with her rapist. Sinclair Lewis's first novel after winning the 1930 Nobel Prize, *Ann Vickers* (1932), was a best-seller about a social worker who gets pregnant after an affair with an army officer, only to go experience the trauma of an abortion when she realizes that the officer does not love her. She then marries a solid but dull fellow, but, to spice things up, has an affair with a judge that leaves her pregnant. Faced with this problem again, she decides to leave her husband to live with the judge. *Ann Vickers* took some of the themes first explored in *Sister Carrie* into a different dimension. The discussion of abortion was considered particularly shocking.

While the movies and literature led the revolt against Victorian morality among the middle classes, a peculiar new genre—the sex confession magazine—made a significant contribution. Pre-eminent in this field was Bernarr Macfadden, who since the 1890s had been the publisher of the journal *Physical Culture*. This was much more than a muscle magazine; it was a guide for living. Macfadden advised "health, vim, and vigor" and all-round physical fitness. Yet there was always something shady about the journal. Models, both men and women, posed nearly naked, fair game for the voyeur. In 1905 Macfadden held the first American female beauty contest in New Jersey. By 1910 the censors had caught up with him and he fled to Brighton, England, where he found solace and a new wife at this sleazy seaside resort and even set up a British version of *Physical Culture*. But his greatest success lay ahead of him upon his return to the United States. In 1919 he started *True Story* magazine, which rapidly became one of the great publishing phenomena in American history. Macfadden had realized that there was a market for romantic stories, and he presented them in the style of the movies as morality tales. "How Life's Lessons Came to Me," "Suppose Your Husband Did This?" and "The Fickleness of Men" were typical. And the success of *True Story* gave rise to such imitators as *True Romances* and *Snappy Stories.*

But the vision of romance that these magazines offered was far removed from that of the Victorians. Love, once mysterious, ethereal, spiritual, even sacred, was suddenly sexualized in a violent way. Thus in "The Fickleness of Men" the hero grabs the heroine: "I snatched her into my arms and held her as in a vise. I smothered her face with my kisses. I was madly infatuated, infatuated beyond vision or hope. . . . I thrust her from me, tingling in every atom of my being." Love became violent infatuation. It was even confused with rape: "Desperately, I tried to keep my senses, everything was going black. 'Do I have to chloroform you or will you promise not to scream' a not unpleasing but firm voice asked," in one story. The heroine here marries the man and declares coyly at the end that "Now we are the lovingest family."

Advertisers too now spread similar ideas. Victorian advertising had generally been made up of photography and drawn captions featuring women in crinolines or bustles, with men always bearded. They were largely concerned with explaining the usefulness of products that people needed. Although ads invariably appeared on the front pages of newspapers, the volume of advertising and the dollars invested in it were far less than today. Although ads sought to entice—especially those for patent medicines—their main intent was to provide information.

In the early twentieth century, though, the techniques and goals of advertising changed beyond recognition. The volume of ads increased sevenfold, spurred by new technology. Advertisers now urged consumers to buy goods not so much because they needed them, but more often as therapy and relief from dull lives. Purchase the product and, consumers were assured, nirvana awaited. Hence around 1900 the voluptuous Gibson Girl replaced dull Victorian images, and after 1915 the flapper and fraternity boy appeared. Ads containing these stereotypes aimed particularly at a burgeoning youth market with spare cash, or appealed to older Americans who yearned to stay young. More dubiously, they promised sexual fulfillment as therapy and gratification if the product were purchased.

Many products could easily be linked to sexual desire. Advertisers of cigarettes, in particular, readily made the association between the use of their product and sexual fulfillment: "When it's the night of the season's festive dance—and Mimi, herself, has consented to go—when in a last moment before starting you thank your good fortune—have a Camel!" Lucky Strike tobacco would not be outdone: "A glassy pond/A red-cheeked maid/And, mingling with the frosty air/the rich relish of Lucky Strike." Spalding swimming suits played very obviously on male fears of sexual failure: "The good old swimming days are here. Oh Boy. But it's great to rip off your shirt, into your suit and splash. But what a shock to some of the poor girls when they see their heroes come out with flat chests and skinny arms, instead of the big husky frames they expected to see. YOU ARE OUT OF LUCK. You are just plain out of luck. Don't try to make excuses. It's your own fault. You can't blame anyone but yourself. But what are you going to do? She's going to find you out." In their urge to sell products, advertisers managed to make even the most unlikely situations sexual. In a 1928 issue of *Good Housekeeping*, an ad for Drano declared that "Every waste pipe faithfully freeflowing—every day of the year." So far, so good; but the ad showed a naked woman, albeit with a towel placed decoratively over her shoulder, yet still revealing hips, buttocks, and back. The subliminal association was evident: even Drano was sexy! The very process of buying things and consuming them was sexy!

There was more. Listerine, which before 1920 was simply an antiseptic for cuts and bruises, became a cure for "halitosis." The invention of this disease of "bad breath" was the hub of one of the 1920s most successful advertising campaigns. If a woman rejected a man's advances, he was told to "suspect yourself first."

It is difficult to overestimate the importance of advertising in the sexualization of American society. Ads promised Americans the satisfaction of their desires—but only temporarily. There was always a new product to buy, always a new desire to be satisfied.

One historian has noted the "greater expectations" of sexual felicity in marriage in the 1910s. Growing material comforts suggested that the struggle for financial survival that had often kept men and women together in the past no longer applied. Couples had the leisure and energy to concentrate on their sexual lives. To meet this demand there appeared in the 1920s a genre of "experts" who published a wide range of newly explicit marriage manuals. Many of the writers had been bohemians in the teens. Widely known as "sex" manuals, sex in these works moved to the forefront of the marriage experience and indeed of all human experience. As Robert and Frances Binkley put it in 1929 in *What Is Right with Marriage*: "The act of sex is appropriately the central fact in the psychological situation of marriage, for in the act a complete system of domestic behavior, both active and passive, can be anticipated." In keeping with this notion there developed "the cult of mutual orgasm," which the marriage manuals of the 1920s and 1930s stressed as the key to health: "the physiological conditions of a normal sex life have the greatest beneficial effect on the whole system." As one manual writer asked, "Can any marriage anchored to this solid bedrock of unsuppressed voluptuous sexual variety fail to become stronger?"

The Dutch writer Theodore van de Velde, in *Ideal Marriage* (1929), a best-selling manual even through the 1960s, provided the first detailed discussion of the technique necessary to attain mutual orgasm. His topics included "love play," "the love-bite," "significance of erogenous zones," and the "genital kiss."

The 1920s saw such a flurry of manuals that in 1929 James Thurber and E. B. White wrote a spoof, *Is Sex Necessary?*, in which the protagonist, confused by all the advice about sex, decides to abandon sex altogether. In the 1960s, the sociologists Dennis Brisset and Lionel S. Lewis dubbed these manuals examples of the work ethic interfering with the process of sex. So it was that sex for men and women became onerous and burdensome: "sex as work." Yet the marriage manuals continued as a hugely popular genre. More explicitly than the movies, literature, advertising, they advised that sex was good for health—which touched a nerve with Americans—even as they whittled away the sense of privacy and the cherished Victorian idea that sex was a natural process.

The 1920s have often been portrayed as an era when the modern oppression of homosexuals grew in severity. The truth is much more complex. In many parts of the United States and the world (for in Weimar Germany there was unprecedented tolerance of homosexuality), the decade was something of a golden age for gays. The historian George Chauncey, Jr., has described a rich urban underworld in New York that by the 1920s had become so vast that it was a highly visible and rich element of the city's culture. Bernarr Macfadden, as early as 1904, had referred with contempt to "the shoals of painted, perfumed, kohl-eyed, lisping, mincing youths that at night swarm on Broadway in the Tenderloin section, or haunt the parks and Fifth Avenue, ogling every man that passes and, it is pleasant to relate, occasionally getting a sound thrashing or an emphatic kicking." By the teens, another New Yorker noted that "our streets and beaches are overrun by . . . fairies." After the war, the cities' trash tabloids frequently made fun of "fairy" attempts to make pickups in the parks and in the elaborate network of gay bathhouses that dotted the cities.

Although New York is not America, evidence is now appearing of similarly vital gay enclaves in Chicago (the red-tie boys), Philadelphia, and other large American cities. And homosexual visibility was promoted by the emerging mass media. One of the first films ever made, in 1895, was of two men dancing a waltz: *The Gay Brothers*. Douglas Fairbanks, Sr., developed his macho image by setting himself up against an imagined homoerotic other. In *Wild and Woolly* (1917), for example, Fairbanks, playing a railway mogul's son, yearns for the countryside in order to get away from the "pansy" world of city life. In *The Mollycoddle* (1920), Fairbanks played an American expatriate living in Europe who has lost touch with his true rugged self. Many more overt implications of homosexuality could be found in the early silent films. Fatty Arbuckle, for example, dabbled in female impersonation in a number of movies such as *Miss Fatty's Seaside Lovers* and *Fatty at Coney Island* (both from 1917). In two films Harold Lloyd toyed with homoerotic themes. In *Grandma's Boy* (1922), two boys sitting on a park bench think they are holding the hand of a girl who is sitting between them, only to discover to their horror that they are in fact holding each other's hands. Lloyd used a similar device in *The Kid Brother* (1927). Here he takes a young woman home. His brothers each think they are inching closer to her, believing she is sleeping behind a curtain. As they manage to touch her, they discover that "she" is Lloyd. But it took Cecil B. DeMille to bring more overt homosexuality into the cinema. His *Salome* (1923), for example, contained a very open homosexual relationship between two Syrian soldiers.

The literature of the 1920s, however, revealed the strongest obsession with homosexuality. The most moving example is Sherwood Anderson's *Winesburg, Ohio* (1919). One of the stories in the book, "Hands," seems to be about a Pennsylvania schoolmaster who is driven out of town because of suspicions that he has homosexual inclinations. F. Scott Fitzgerald used several homosexual characters to set off his more virile ones. In *Tender Is the Night* (1934) the monocled Campion succeeds "somehow to restrain his most blatant effeminacy." Sinclair Lewis in *Dodsworth* (1929) has the German, Kurt, take strait-laced Sam Dodsworth into a Berlin gay bar. In Ludwig Lewisohn's *Stephen Escott* (1930), a lengthy discussion speculates that if women were to abdicate their role as uplifters of men, it would lead to more homosexuality: "There is a distinct increase in homosexuality already," Lewisohn declared fearfully.

Sex and marriage manuals were similarly concerned with homosexuality. The bohemian Clement Wood, in *Manhood: The Facts of Life Presented to Men* (1924), went so far as to calculate the percentage of adolescent male desire that was homoerotic. To this point, the vast amount of discussion of homosexuality drew on earlier, even Victorian, ideas about the frequenters of the urban underworld as essentially sad and effeminate creatures, objects of pity. But different agendas reflected a growing confusion about the development of homosexual identity and ultimately subverted the middle-class male world of romantic friendship. A growing body of work suggested that homosexuality need not be confined to an underworld of effeminate degenerates. Horrifyingly, one could now easily be identified as a homosexual. Joseph Collins, in his best-selling *The Doctor Looks at Love and Life* (1926), took up this theme: "There are many persons who indulge in unnatural sexual relations who are not homosexuals. They are the real degenerates. There are many potential and actual homosexuals whose intercourse with members of their own sex is confined to emotional and intellectual contact, to establishing romantic friendship." Homosexuals might be everywhere!

What now became of Victorian male romantic friendship? What now of Christian brotherhood? A key tenet of how American males understood one another had been placed under suspicion. In some quarters this stirred up a crisis in masculinity as great as that at the turn of the century. A dramatic scandal at the naval base in Newport, Rhode Island, in 1919, when a vast network of homosexuals was uncovered, epitomized this crisis. Shockingly, a local Episcopalian minister, Samuel Kent, was accused of engaging in sexual activity with a number of homosexual men. Kent vehemently denied this, insisting that his interest in the men was purely brotherly in the Victorian tradition. He was excused, but the Victorian male world of romantic friendship was clearly now suspect. What young men did together could now no longer be innocent.

The female world of love and ritual escaped more intact despite a growing awareness of lesbianism in the 1920s. The teens had seen the development of a lesbian club in Greenwich Village, Heterodoxy. Here a number of bohemian women explored their lesbian potential. They neatly complemented the network of lesbian bars that dotted Greenwich Village. The appearance of Edouard Bourdet's *The Captive* on Broadway in 1926, however, attained international publicity and, according to the historian Jonathan Katz, "marked a historical turning point in the middle-class public's awareness of women-to-women love." Much of the controversy produced by the play was because at its conclusion, the leading lady left her man for a woman who never appeared on stage. This obviously upset a great many men, who could fear that the same might happen to them.

Even more influential in making lesbianism culturally visible, and thus drawing an element of suspicion into women's romantic friendship, was the furor over Radclyffe Hall's *The Well of Loneliness* (1928). The subject of a celebrated court case in Britain, the book dealt openly with the struggles of the heroine, Stephen Gordon, to come to terms with her lesbian desires. When the work was seized by the New York police, a debate followed in the pages of America's leading journals. In the *New Republic*, Robert Lovett concluded that there was "something to be said for the view that the normal must be kept from knowledge of the invert lest the latter infect the former."

The cult of "slumming," which became vogue in America in the 1920s, smoothed the spread of underworld ideas. The novelist Carl Van Vechten led the way in his 1925 exploration of life in Harlem, *Nigger Heaven*. The message implied in the novel was that white culture was too repressed by comparison with African-American culture. In the novel, the editor Ronald Durwood observes that whites on Long Island enjoy the same things as the blacks of Harlem, "but it is vastly more amusing than the Long Island set for the simple reason that [the blacks are] amused." When Van Vechten arranged for two black entertainers to visit Mabel Dodge Luhan's salon, it was too much even for her. "They both leered and rolled their suggestive eyes and made me feel first hot then cold," she exclaimed. A whole genre of American writing in the 1920s drew on the writers' experience of the underworld. For Waldo Frank, black men were "big fellows with flourishing moustaches, bushy brows. They are obscene with brutal energy." Sherwood Anderson, who joined in the vogue, referred to the "slender flanks like running horses—bodies like young Gods" of New Orleans' African Americans. A popular song urged people to "go inspectin'" "like Carl Van Vechten." And many of the middle-class young did just that.

In the 1920s, youth enjoyed freedoms that they had never before imagined possible. The New Freedom was even more striking for young middle-class women who had jobs and spare money and the freedom to go out on dates without chaperones. This was the New Woman or "flapper" who has become one of the great symbols of American culture in the 1920s, and who continued to claim the benefits of the advances in women's roles that had begun before the war. F. Scott Fitzgerald romanticized her as "lovely and expensive and about nineteen." But she aroused the ire of moralists. The president of the University of Florida railed at the "low-cut gowns, the rolled hose and short skirts [that] are born of the Devil and his angels, and are carrying the present and future generations to chaos and destruction." The flapper drank even as drinking was illegal; she indulged in the "filthy" habit of smoking; and she might swear. Worse, she was quite prepared to be frank and brazen about her sexual activities, huffing and puffing that she suffered from "sex starvation" and avidly reading Freud. The historian Kenneth Yellis put it best: "What was being challenged was the Victorian conception of sexuality and the roles of men and women."

The continued rise of the "flapper" was symptomatic of much deeper changes in the experience and meaning of courtship among Americans. These changes reflected the greater importance of youth in American society and the greater freedoms granted to the young. As urbanization and industrialization advanced, youth found themselves less bound by community strictures. With more money in their pockets, they became primary targets for the new leisure industries. Movie theatres, amusement parks, and dance halls, which in the early years of the century had been frequented primarily by the working class, now became the site of middle-class courtship. And by the 1920s the automobile had established it-self as a major catalyst in enhancing youth's freedoms.

With so much more of society geared to their every whim, young people took the opportunity to indulge. It was scarcely surprising that traditional Victorian patterns of courtship began to break down. Young people simply no longer needed to bother about the formalities of "calling"; and they certainly didn't need to worry about a maiden aunt acting as a chaper-one. All a young man had to do was to call a girl on the tele-phone and ask her for a "date." By the late 1920s the "dating system" had replaced the Victorian system of courtship.

On its surface the "dating system"—unaccompanied dates —seems far more like conformity than youthful rebellion. The development of the institution of dating entailed a mov-ing away of courtship from the firm guidance of the older generation to control by a peer-led youth culture with its own way of enforcing its codes. The morality of their peers was ef-fective in keeping young people in line because the threat of being shown up and losing out in the "popularity" contest tuned in with youth's deepest fears of rejection. Hence the rit-uals of what the sociologist Willard Waller called the "rating and dating complex" developed in America's high schools and colleges. Young men and women had to struggle to keep up their rating in this competitive game. For example, a young man had to cultivate a "line" to try to convince the girl that he had "fallen seriously in love with her." The boy and girl "each tried to make the other fall in love by pretending that they had not already done so." Waller dubbed this "the principle of least interest"—he or she who was least bothered about the continuation of the relationship had the upper hand. What could be more conformist?

Despite these conservative aspects, the dating game repre-sented a rebellion against Victorianism that subverted tradi-tional morality because of its built-in cynicism: it injected into

personal life the rough and tumble of the public world. The
"rating and dating complex" became a new departure that
heralded an era of conflict in social relations between the
sexes. Where Victorian courtship had tended to be a serious
matter with marriage as its goal, "rating and dating" was a period of fun and frolics that might last for years before engagement and marriage were decided. The possibilities for
ambiguity and misunderstanding were limitless. And the opportunities for mutual exploitation in the search for "thrills"
boundless.

Sex and money featured heavily in these hostilities. "The
Too High Cost of Courting" upset one young man in 1924
who claimed that he had recently spent more than three hundred dollars on women, to no avail. After all, men expected a
good return on their investment. Thus women should permit
a little petting. If they did not, men might accuse them of
being "gold diggers." The problem of the low return on the
cost of a date was a feature of numerous magazine articles: "I
Hatem" wrote to the adviser-to-the-lovelorn of the *St. Louis
Post Dispatch* declaring that "City girls are all gold-diggers
and deceivers." "John" in New York complained that "a certain young lady who accepts my gifts has a habit of disap-
pointing me on the night of the date. Should I continue to go
with her?"

Sex became the greatest source of argument. A major topic
of discussion among youth centered on how far it was permissible to go while "dating." Where were the boundaries? What
did the new morality of the youth culture prescribe? Unlike
their hippy grandchildren, 1920s youth debated whether to go
all the way, but few did. Their concerns were with "petting."
The term was new in the 1920s; related words that delineated
similar physical practices, such as "necking," "spooning," and
even "snuggle-pupping," still had currency. "Petting" could
describe any sexual stimulation beyond mere kissing, clothed

or unclothed—that is, "the necks, lips and ears utilized extensively as sexual objects." Or it could include "literally every caress known to married couples," falling short of sexual intercourse. The term became a vague, ill-defined, all-inclusive bogeyman. But the petting fad made noncoital relationships overtly sexual among middle-class youth who had no intention of getting married because it worked, not as a preliminary to the sex act but as a "pseudo-substitute for it, as a means of working off tense emotions." Kinsey's figures indicate that petting to climax was indeed on the increase. Before World War I, 29 percent of girls petted; ten years later, 43 percent. There were similar figures for boys in these years: a rise from 41 to 51 percent in numbers who petted to climax. Petting was positively accepted as a key part of what the peer-led youth culture recommended. As one wag noted, "Since petting leads to 'dates' and 'dates' lead to more 'dates' and to real romance, one must pet or be left behind."

Yet the term's vagueness was symptomatic of a confused time of change. The hedonism of popular culture had influenced behavior, but cultural lag ensured that older values persisted. Youth commented on the "many mores" that were available to them. The social commentator Theodore Newcomb observed that "It is expected by both boys and girls that men should prefer virginity in girls, but don't insist"; "Boys do not expect nor particularly want the Victorian concept of purity in the girl they marry"; "It is right and decent to have intimate relations with the person you love, but you mustn't be promiscuous—that's cheap and vulgar." It was not quite the case that, as the contemporary song went, "Heaven knows, anything goes." But in some circles most anything did. And with family and religion increasingly taking a back seat to what went on in the rumble seat of the automobile, sexual values changed rapidly. The Lynds, visiting Middletown in the early 1920s, observed that "a heavy taboo supported by law

and by both religion and popular sanctions, rests on sexual relations between persons who are not married." Returning in
the mid-1930s for *Middletown in Transition* (revealingly subti-
tled *A Study in Cultural Conflicts*), they discovered that "the
range of sanctions is wider, the definition of the one 'right
way' less clear, causing confusion." Flaming youth had replaced an official Victorian single standard of qualified
chastity before marriage, and an unofficial double standard by
which this did not apply to men, with a single standard that
permitted varying degrees of sexual pleasure—petting—between young men and women on a date. As the Spanish
writer Ortega y Gasset summed up the direction in which
things were heading: "The old immorality has become the
new morality."

The consequence of this confusion and doubt over shifting
moral values and gender roles were tensions between the
sexes. While heated debates in Victorian journals had articu-
lated men's and women's complaints about each other, the
tone had always been respectful. Now the mood was quite different. Both sexes saw each other as competitive. High school
girls chided men in the high school newspaper: "Boys, is it fair
to make the girls come to a school entertainment unescorted?
So far, I have not been to an entertainment without seeing
three-fourths of the girls come without escorts. The most disgusting thing about it is that boys act as though they did not
realize the predicament they've placed the girls in. . . ." Girls
wrote openly to advice columnists to complain about their boyfriends as "cads," "sheiks," and "bounders." There was far
worse: the actress Gloria Swanson was quoted as saying that
"the more I see of men, the more I like dogs." Men hit back at
this kind of stereotyping. Young men had bull sessions in college to discuss the antics of flappers, who they described as
"chickens." Hence movie starlets were "beautiful, but dumb."

Girls wrote to advice columnists to complain about "smutty" comments that their boyfriends might make. The sociologist Ernest Burgess noted that sex now was "an open subject and repartee for discussion among mixed groups." Another commentator noted that "Sex was as widely discussed as mothballs."

By the late 1920s Greenwich Village and underworld styles of morality had begun to influence the mainstream. This was perhaps best exemplified by the rise of "companionate marriage." This was not the same as the sociological term that refers to the trend toward nonpatriarchal marriage after 1850. Rather, "companionate marriage" was a concoction of the reformer Judge Ben Lindsey of the juvenile courts of Denver, Colorado. Looking to his experience of the working class of that city, he noted their tendency to cohabit before marriage. Worrying too about the divorce rate, he recommended a kind of marriage whereby it was possible to divorce at any time before the birth of children. This was trial marriage. If marriage could be so easily dissolved, couples would surely end theirs at the slightest sign of difficulty. Companionate marriage was a fad that actually attracted a great deal of attention at the time. Conservatives lambasted Lindsey for the threat he posed to the family. The Episcopal bishop of New York City declared the book "one of the most filthy . . . pieces of propaganda ever published on behalf of lewdness, promiscuity, adultery, and unrestrained sexual gratification." Many couples even tried it—then, of course, divorced. Despite its faddishness, its significance should not be underestimated: it was a direct assault on an institution that Victorians regarded as sacrosanct, and it looked ahead toward cohabitation and the contract marriages of the 1960s.

Women's greater expectations of marriage contributed to the increase in divorce during the 1920s. One woman com-

plained in her divorce suit that her husband refused "reasonable and natural" intercourse, which had "resulted in a serious
and permanent impairment of her health." Another woman
expected to be in love and stay in love with the man she married. One woman in her divorce petition declared, "There is
nothing doing, your efforts are hopeless. I have lost all affection for you. I can live with whomsoever I please at any time,
provided I have sufficient love for him and I have no love for
you. All is over between us. You do not fit my ideal of a man."

The rising divorce rate, a seven-fold increase between the
1880s and 1920s, alarmed traditionalists. In 1928 one in six
marriages ended in divorce, making it an important issue in
the 1920s, widely discussed in all sorts of magazines. Periodi-
cal literature contained articles from hurt spouses, such as
"End of the Trail by a Bewildered Husband" in *Sunset*. Such
accounts are distressing to read, even today. Yet divorce became big business in the 1920s. Reno, Nevada, became the nation's divorce capital. Nevada, with a shrewd eye for the main
chance, insisted on a six-week residency, but in return divorce
would be instantaneous and easy. Gambling joints appeared to
amuse those fulfilling the residency requirement. The rest of
the country savored tales of the goings-on in Reno. Gradually
divorce became routinized. The Lynds noted the impact of the
rising divorce rate: "Marriage need not be final, since divorce
is no longer a serious disgrace." Divorce challenged Victorian
morality not just because Victorians had not approved of it,
but because divorce made marriage—the very heart of Victorian morality—less sacred.

Thus by the end of the twenties, most of the key tenets of
the shift from Victorian morality were in place: a media
geared to profit, and an urban middle class that soaked up the
liberated messages of popular culture and whose youth lacked
the moral fiber to resist the temptations of consumption and
leisure. To these people Victorian morality seemed increas-

ingly an anomaly. Dating and petting, companionate marriage, and easier divorce set the agenda for the twentieth century. Now, however, the new morality was to be tested by the most serious economic distress in the nation's history.

4

From Depression to War

IN OCTOBER 1929 the New York stock market crashed. There followed the greatest economic crisis in American history. Within months, the free and liberated style of living that the prosperity of the 1920s had fueled seemed out of tune with an economy now in freefall.

Both middle- and working-class Americans now faced a struggle to survive. By 1932, unemployment in the workforce—just 3.2 percent in 1929—had reached 23.6 percent. In the circumstances, Americans found themselves battling for their basic needs. By 1933, Americans on average had only 54 percent of the income they had enjoyed in 1929. In the year 1932 no less than 28 percent of the households in the country had no income at all from regular employment. This problem was widespread. Half the workforce in Cleveland was without a job at the height of the depression, while at one point the figure for Toledo was as high as 80 percent. Although among the industrialized nations Germany suffered most, the United States suffered longest: it is now agreed that only the tremendous boost to production that came with World War II brought the United States out of the Great Depression.

The effects on social and moral life were enormous. The 1920s party came abruptly to a halt as the Victorian producer and self-help ethic revived strongly. But after President Franklin Roosevelt inaugurated his series of dramatic New

Deal reforms in 1933, while the depression did not end, consumer demand grew as a firm national market was reestablished. This created a greater sense of security than in the early 1930s, and some of the social trends of the twenties then resumed. They were reinforced by a mood of recklessness, a sense of living for the here-and-now, and a willingness to take chances that seemed to be a product of the depression's fear and uncertainty. But Americans also felt a cautious dependence on tradition. As a consequence both the revolt against Victorian morality and the repression of alternative sexualities by traditionalists gained pace in these tense years.

As the courts grappled with the issue of obscenity in the 1930s, their decisions significantly extended the bounds of sexual expression. The first important legal case arose out of the permission in the 1930 Tariff Act to "admit the so-called classics or books of recognized and established literary or scientific merit" as an exception from the law against the importation of pornography. Random House publishers decided to test this provision when a copy of the work they intended to publish—James Joyce's *Ulysses*—was seized by U.S. customs. After deliberation, Judge John M. Woolsey declared the Irish novel an "amazing tour de force" that "does not excite sexual impulses or lustful thoughts in a person with average sex instincts" and therefore was outside the American legal system's definition of obscenity as "tending to stir the sex impulses or lead to sexually impure or lustful thoughts." Woolsey called in two literary assessors to confirm that, like him, they felt the book to be "a somewhat tragic and very powerful commentary on the inner lives of men and women." No wonder the 1934 Modern Library edition of *Ulysses* described the decision as a great triumph against "Puritanism": "the first week of December 1933 will go down in history for two repeals, that of prohibition and that of the legal compulsion for squeamishness in literature."

The second significant case, *People v. Viking Press*, concerned the work of an American author, Erskine Caldwell's *God's Little Acre* (1933), a novel of Southern rural life, which was accused of obscenity. A New York City magistrate named Greenspan mused that writers experienced the same difficulties as sex reformers: how could they go about their work by using nonobscene language? Greenspan sympathized with Caldwell's efforts to describe the "sex side of life" and Caldwell's publisher's insistence on the "high literary merit" of his work. Greenspan declared that "there is no way of anticipating [a book's] effect upon a disordered or diseased mind, and if the courts were to exclude books from sale merely because they might incite lust in disordered minds, our entire literature might be reduced to a small number of relatively uninteresting and barren books." As the historian Rochelle Gurstein has recently noted, "This was a direct rebuttal of the position that public morals and decency took precedence over literary culture." The experts had spoken. The floodgates had been opened.

Yet attitudes toward censorship reflected the ambiguity about sexual morality that typified the decade. Book censorship encouraged the revolt. Yet censorship gained ground in the movies. The new "talkies" enjoyed an era of experimentation and openness that they were not to have again for many decades. At the depression's onset, several films were passed for general release that simply would not have been later in the decade. Movies, after all, provided escape from difficult lives. In particular, the films of Marlene Dietrich and Greta Garbo caused an uproar. In *Blue Angel* (1930), Dietrich plays a cabaret singer who has a torrid affair with a repressed professor. In *Blond Venus* (1932) she sleeps with Cary Grant to obtain money for her dying husband, who rejects her after finding out. She is forced to become a prostitute, which energizes her sufficiently to return eventually to her recovered husband.

Greta Garbo in *Susan Lenox: Her Rise and Fall* (1932) plays a farm girl of Swedish-American extraction. She has an affair with Clark Gable, which ends when she begins a relationship with a carnival proprietor. She goes on to have a number of liaisons with wealthy men, but she realizes that she still loves Gable, whom she follows around desperately pleading for forgiveness.

Perhaps the best example of the openness of the pictures that preceded the movies' self-imposed production code was Garbo's *Queen Christina* (1933). This film was based on the life of a seventeenth-century Swedish queen who enjoyed dressing as a man. While out one day she meets and falls for the envoy of the Spanish king, who is bringing a proposal of marriage. She falls in love with the envoy and abdicates her throne to be with him before he is killed in a duel. The film was notable for its cross-dressing and its portrayal of a woman with strong sexual feelings.

Garbo and Dietrich flourished in the early 1930s, perhaps because they were European. Mae West, however, was to prove too much provocation for Hollywood. Paramount decided that *Diamond Lil* would make a blockbuster film. This proposal, however, arrived at a very difficult time in the history of the movies. The possibilities of the talkie redefined the fierce debate over censorship. Moralists feared that actors could now justify and explain their behavior. A crisis blew up when New York and Chicago adopted strong censorship codes. In 1929 a group of Roman Catholics, prominent among whom were Martin Quigley and Timothy Breen, had set up the Legion of Decency which proposed a new means of controlling the movies. As a result, in 1930 a code was adopted to censor the movies. Devised by the reformer Daniel Lord, it set forth the principle that films should not be permitted to create "sympathy" for amoral behavior. If corruption were to be portrayed, it must be clear that it was wrong and that "good [is] right." With surprising speed, Hollywood executives accepted the code on principle, but it was uncertain how binding it would be.

When he heard that West's play was being considered for a movie by rival Paramount, Harry Warner of Warner Bros. wrote to Will Hays, head of the Motion Picture Producers and Distributors of America: "Please wire immediately whether I can believe my ears that Paramount has arranged to make *Diamond Lil* with Mae West. . . . Recollect that it was absolutely definite that *Diamond Lil* was not to be produced. . . . I am not sending this wire as a protest but I want to know how to run our business in future." West could be a hot property at the box office in a time of declining movie revenues brought on by the depression. In 1932 Paramount was facing a $21 million loss. In a compromise of sorts, *Diamond Lil* was filmed as *She Done Him Wrong*. Yet as the movie trade journal *Variety* indicated, "Nothing much has changed except the title." James Wingate, director of the Studio Relations Department at Paramount, noted that "West gives a performance of strong realism." In the face of West's popularity, there was nothing the censors could do: the voluntary code lacked teeth. The film was an enormous success, breaking box office records nationally and internationally.

West's follow-up, *I'm No Angel* (1933), extended the West persona. Her innuendos flew thick and fast: "When I'm good, I'm very good. When I'm bad, I'm better." When the West character Tira is accused of "knowing" a number of men, she declares, "It's not the men in my life, but the life in my men." Martin Quigley, a strong lay Catholic as well as publisher of the trade journal *Exhibitor's Herald World,* commented on the film, "There is no more pretense here of romance than there is on a stud farm." Critic Joseph Wood Krutch branded West "simple-minded, lurid and crude." But the shocks of moralists did not affect her popularity.

West's success, however, was not to last. Pressure had been growing to apply the production code more stringently, not just because of West's films but because of a whole burst of other "sex films." West, however, was the prime target of the much more effective 1934 Production Code. It included a number of rules for the presentation of sex: "Impure love must not be presented as attractive and beautiful" and, almost with West in mind, "it must not be the subject of comedy or farce, or treated as material for laughter." West's career nosedived. Her next film, *It Ain't No Sin* (1934), did not attract as many moviegoers because it was not nearly as provocative as her others. She then fought voraciously to film *Klondike Annie* (1936) with the innuendo that had made her famous. But it could not save her career. By 1940 she was reduced to playing in the comedy *My Little Chickadee,* which, while it revived a stereotype of the older West persona, was so boring that it bombed at the box office.

West had gone too far carrying the 1920s flapper type to its logical conclusion and presenting a woman character who was truly brazen, sexual, and assertive. The powerful champions of traditional moral values in American society—in large part through her provocation—now reasserted themselves in a manner that challenged and limited artistic freedom.

After the 1934 code the exploration of risqué themes became exceedingly difficult for filmmakers. There was to be no more revealing clothing for women, and, famously, even married couples were to be shown in twin, not double, beds. To be sure, numerous roles for strong women, albeit devoid of overt sexual content, now appeared, such as Scarlett O'Hara in *Gone with the Wind* (1939) and Bette Davis in *Dangerous* (1935) and *Jezebel* (1938). And there were many roles for career women, notably in the films of Joan Crawford, who played a cub reporter in *Dance, Fools, Dance* (1931), a stenographer in *Grand Hotel* (1932), and a cabaret singer in *The Bride Wore Red*

(1937). But the mid-1930s success of Shirley Temple symbolized how far Hollywood had been stunted by the code. As a child before the age of puberty, her innocence was not in doubt. And to prove it, when the English author Graham Greene noted in an article her appeal to pedophiles, Temple's outraged studio sued.

It is no coincidence that the censorship of Hollywood films reached its peak in the 1934 production code. In a time of great national insecurity, the devisers of the code acknowledged the public need for a return to moral certainties. Hollywood dutifully fell into line. In an era of economic meltdown, if moviemakers were not allowed to sell sex they had better sell sexual morality.

In the same mood, the 1930s saw the suppression of America's burgeoning gay community. In New York City the police launched harassment campaigns against clubs that included "pansy" acts in their itinerary and against the city's drag balls. The aim was to return the homosexual community to the confines of the Village and Harlem; gay people were even driven out of their outdoors gathering places. Ironically the repeal of prohibition, which had done so much to help the growth of gay bars in the 1920s, led directly to their suppression in the 1930s. The New York State Liquor Authority, established to license alcohol sales, decided it would sell to no establishment that was not "orderly." The SLA in its wisdom deemed that gay bars were not "orderly," and it determined to make full use of its power to deny licenses. Over the twenty-five years it closed numerous bars, some fully gay or lesbian and others merely gay-friendly.

Together with the shutting down of bars, the early depression years saw renewed censorship of the representation of homosexuality. State legislatures forbade plays from "depicting or dealing with the subject of sex degeneracy, or sex perversion." Playwrights simply were banned from any discussion of homosexuality. In February 1931 the RKO vaudeville circuit banned its performers from using words like "fairy" and "pansy" in their acts; while the initial Hollywood Production Code of 1930, which had tolerated discussion of adultery and murder with a moral point, absolutely excluded discussion of homosexuality. Thus a clear atmosphere of repression pervaded the early depression years as Americans reached for the familiar in an uncertain world.

In the early 1930s, as Americans reined in their resources, marriage, divorce, and birthrates all fell quickly. The bleak economic times had an especially profound impact on couples' engagements. The meaning of engagement became much more ambiguous as couples were forced to stay engaged and put off marriage for longer and longer periods because of a shortage of money. The marriage rate of 10.14 per thousand persons in 1929 fell to 7.87 per thousand by 1932. According to one estimate, by 1938, 1.5 million people had been forced to delay marriage. One counselor speculated that "the natural hopes of an [engaged] couple are frustrated . . . they are likely to feel rebellious against a social system that they hold responsible for their disappointment." One young man who had to wait four years before marrying his fiancée pleaded to an advice columnist: "But gosh, nature never meant the preliminaries to last so long! Nature never intended the courtship to be dragged out forever. . . ." Another remembered, "I was engaged for a long time, but I couldn't get a job." A young college graduate clerk in Middletown on ten dollars a week declared, "I'm stuck. There's just no future for our generation, and there's nothing I can do about it. I don't expect to marry—I can't." A leading marriage counselor urged the young to shorten their engagements: "In Heaven's name, why wait [for marriage]? . . . If you are sincerely in love, old enough to know what you are doing . . . you have no right to let anything, least of all money, bar you from happiness." But as a schoolteacher, Elsa Ponselle, noted, some brief delays of marriage became permanent. Writing decades later she asked, "Do you realize how many people in my generation are not married? . . . It wasn't that we didn't have a chance. I was going with someone when the depression hit. We would probably have gotten married. He was a commercial artist. . . . Suddenly, he was laid off. It hit him like a ton of bricks. And he just disappeared." In 1935 the proportion of single women unmarried between twenty-five and thirty was 30 percent higher than it had been five years earlier.

Hence the growing array of marriage guidance experts that appeared during the decade began to adjust the ritual of engagement to the new conditions. Their solution was to suggest that it become less of a commitment toward a permanent marriage. Betrothal, which until recently had been rare to break, now became a further time of testing one another's personalities and sexual compatibility. Margaret Sanger noted that "the fiancée's breath, odor, touch, embrace and kiss must be pleasing. . . . If they are not . . . then under no circumstances should the engagement be prolonged." The sociologists Ernest Burgess and Paul Wallin, in their major 1930s study *Engagement and Marriage,* noted that "even engagement has become a trial relationship during which love is assessed. . . . It is now considered the last stage in the selection process . . . its preeminent function the final opportunity for the couple to find out if they are fitted for each other."

Once together it seemed that couples stuck at marriage longer. Between 1928 and 1933 the divorce rate of the population dropped 43 percent. In 1932 alone the rate dropped from 1.63 per thousand to 1.28 per thousand. Partly this was because getting on relief was a far simpler process if one was the chief breadwinner for a family. Reflecting the strong revival of a self-help ethos, the Lynds in *Middletown in Transition* reported a newspaper editorial that observed, "Many a family that has lost its car has found its soul." They described the depression as "good for the family."

But at what a cost. For many unemployed men, the impact on their self-respect was devastating. The psychologist Nathan Ackerman recalled: "I did a little field work among the unemployed miners in Pennsylvania. Just observing. What the lack of a job, two, three, four years did to their families and to them. They hung around street corners and in groups. They gave each other solace. They were loath to go home because they were indicted as if it were their fault for being unemployed. A jobless man was a lazy good-for-nothing." Once again the Victorian work ethic affected men. Ackerman continued that "the women punished the men for not bringing home the bacon, by withholding themselves sexually. By belittling and emasculating the men, undermining their parental authority, turning to the eldest son. . . . These men were desperately downcast. They felt despised, they were ashamed of themselves. They cringed, they comforted one another. They avoided home." A bevy of sociological studies appeared confirming observations like Ackerman's that the depression challenged men's status. The most famous of these was the sociologist Mirra Komarovsky's *The Unemployed Man and His Family* (1940), which suggested that the extent of male unemployment and lack of job security had upset gender relations and weakened men's role within the family. As one wife noted, "They're not men anymore, if you know what I mean." The author Meridel Le Sueur commented that "He cannot provide. If he propagates he cannot take care of his young. The means are not in his hands." The depression thus upset the solid, sturdy image of manliness that had been so central to Victorianism.

This anxiety about masculinity was reinforced by a decline in the birthrate, which for the first time fell below the replacement level. From 21.3 births per thousand in 1930, the number dropped to 18.4 per thousand by 1933. Families were putting off having children until they could afford it. Meridel Le Sueur noted women's fears: "I don't want to marry. I don't want any children. So they all say. No children. No marriage."

This significant decline in the birthrate vividly demonstrated the deep consequences of the depression. The greater availability of birth control made it possible. By World War I, dissemination of birth-control literature and devices had become legal in most states. By 1930 the American Birth Control League had fifty-five birth-control clinics throughout the country, but by 1938 there were as many as five hundred. By the end of the decade, as fear of an upsurge in welfare babies grew, the federal government for the first time provided funds for birth control. In 1937 the AMA ceased to oppose it. As early as 1931 the Federal Council of Churches came out in support of contraception. A 1936 Gallup Poll revealed that 63 percent of Americans approved of birth control. Reflecting this, contraceptives were now available from the Sears, Roebuck catalog. In *Middletown* in the mid-1930s a "leading downtown druggist" reported that sales of contraceptives had been steadily increasing over ten years. He did not think there had been any particular increase on account of the depression. But he did notice "more frankness on the part of both sexes in asking for various contraceptive aids." In the 1930s birth control and contraceptives became more common.

The birth-control movement succeeded in part because it opposed abortion. Yet women had abortions in the 1930s on an unprecedented scale. Quite simply, married women who already had children could not afford any more. Those women who were not married could not afford to get married. In 1936 the New Jersey police discovered a Birth Control Club that contained no less than eight hundred members, mostly working-class "clerks." In return for their club fees, they were entitled to regular examinations and surgical procedures as required. A postwar study by the Kinsey Institute concluded that "the depression of the 1930s resulted in a larger proportion of pregnancies that were artificially aborted." Among women born between 1890 and 1919, the highest rate of induced abortion took place "during the depth of the depression." A study by Dr. Regine K. Stix of women visiting a New York City birth control clinic in 1931 and 1932 found a similar pattern. She explained why one young woman terminated her pregnancy—"because she was the breadwinner in the family and could not afford to lose her job, much less produce another mouth to feed." Kinsey's findings even suggest that there may have been a trend toward aborting first pregnancies.

Married African-American women, too, resorted to abortion more often during the depression. Dr. Charles H. Garvin noted in 1932 that among blacks there had occurred "a very definite increase in the numbers of abortions, criminally performed, among the married." In 1935 the Harlem Hospital opened a special ward to treat women who needed care after illegal abortions.

After the decline of the divorce rate in the early 1930s, it began to rise anew in mid-decade. In *Middletown,* divorce continued to cause scandal, yet the citizens' toleration of it grew: "Daily in the courtrooms [their] businessmen lawyers work in the matter-of-fact spirit of their world of contractual relations." They cited a lawyer who declared that "marriage is a contract and that anyone twenty-one years old ought to be able to get out of it just about as easily as he gets into it." So much for Victorian ideas of the sanctity of marriage. Many other Middletowners paid only lip service to marriage: "There is still a great deal of married men's running around with single women here," the Lynds noted. Lawyers confirmed this in several conversations: "Ever since the World War, people here have gotten more free and immoral. A married man used to slip away for a few nights; but now he doesn't mind being seen in the street with another woman, for nobody minds." "Swinging," a practice later to become synonymous with the 1970s, appeared even in the 1930s: "Then there are nowadays these parties where a few young married couples get to drinking together; and one husband makes a cryptic remark to another's wife, and one thing leads to another." By 1935 "infidelity [wasn't] regarded as seriously as formerly." Hence the deep loosening of mores that had begun in the 1920s continued in the 1930s because people's sense of desperation encouraged the breaking of taboos.

This theme persisted in other ways too. Much of the leisure culture of the 1920s declined in the 1930s because of hard economic times and the renewal of repression. But the great amusement parks survived. Their owners focused on advertising at ballrooms and beaches. Coney Island flourished, though it had little fresh investment. Crowds of people still came for a dime round-trip from the city and enjoyed rides and hot dogs for no more than a nickel. In the mid-1930s a vogue for dance marathons also caught the imagination of the public.

The relaxation of mores continued on college campuses and in high schools. *Fortune* magazine in 1937 noted that "Sex is no longer news." The Lynds on their return to Middletown in the mid-1930s noted that the young were "more knowing and bold." The boys regarded necking as part and parcel of a date. "We fellows used occasionally get slapped for doing things, but the girls don't do that much anymore." The Lynds' research did not support the idea of a conservative reaction in the 1930s: "Our High School students of both sexes are increasingly sophisticated. They know everything and do everything—openly. And they aren't ashamed to talk about it." Other observers of America's youth judged the situation similarly. Dorothy Bromley and Florence Britten's study of college students, *Youth and Sex,* from 1938, confirmed the impact of the automobile: "Joe and Jane petting in the back seat of an automobile are unimportant. Five million boys and girls petting on public highways have national significance. They indicate a social revolution in manners and morals. Courtship had left the family roof and taken to the road." But Bromley and Britten believed girls still had matters firmly under control. *Fortune* noted that "half the men and twenty-five percent of the women had indulged in premarital relations." But the sexual partners of college women were usually their fiancés: girls still lacked the sexual freedom of boys. *Fortune* summed up the prevailing ethic of the New Deal era as " 'reasonable restraint,' particularly on the part of the girls, before marriage, and fidelity on both sides after marriage." Although strong challenges to the Victorian ethic continued, the 1930s also represented the beginning of a period of reaction as Americans relished the familiar and traditional; hence the censorship of the movies and the repression of homosexuality. In these years Americans for the most part had their minds on financial survival.

The depression ended not with the triumphant success of the New Deal but with the war. Gross national product, $90 billion in 1939, by 1945 rose to $213 billion. Unemployment all but disappeared while a growing demand for labor placed whole groups previously excluded in a far stronger position in the labor market. The prosperity that arrived with wartime helped bring about a rise in both the marriage rate and the birthrate. Yet anxiety and a sense of foreboding, now caused by the war as well as by memories of the depression, continued as families grew stronger. And the powerful undercurrents of the revolt against Victorian sexual morality still flowed.

War intensified romantic and sexual relationships. Young men who knew they might die were less bothered about moral codes that called for sexual restraint. In Hawaii a

woman who worked in a cafeteria and had seven children remarked that "The Service boys they get into your nerve....
When you serve them, they call you 'Hey, lady, how about a
date. Hey, lady, what are you doing tonight?' They try to have
a date. It doesn't matter who.... The service boys, maybe they
don't mean it. They away from home and they are lonesome."
Although American soldiers in Britain in fact belied their
stereotypical image of being "oversexed and over here," as D
day approached relationships intensified: there was a feeling
that these were the last nights that men and women might
make love, and there was little byplay or persuasion. "People
were for love, so to speak. It was easy to fall in love." One contemporary observer noted that "From officers to privates,
we're obsessed by sex, and much the same seems true of the
civilian population."

This experience was echoed on the home front in the
United States and on the field of battle. The marriage rate accelerated as couples married more readily in better economic
times; and in the heat of the moment the possibility of death
added urgency. One woman said, "I've told him I don't love
him, but he's an aviator and he says I should marry him any-
how and give him a little happiness. He says he knows he'll be
dead in a year." Between 1940 and 1946 three million more
Americans married than might have been expected to had
marriage rates remained the same as before the war. This was
a clear recovery from the lows of the depression. GIs especially
married at the rate of a thousand a day. Many such marriages
in this "rush to the altar" were barely viable and would end in
divorce. One corporal recalled, "I did something stupid, I got
drunk last night and when I woke up and looked down there
was ninety-eight pounds of woman flesh beside me, and
she ... reminded me that we had gotten married. But I don't
want to be married." A woman wrote of her failed marriage
that "You get married and you don't have enough time to re-

ally learn to know each other. . . . But I'm not sorry I married him, and I wouldn't tell other girls not to marry like I did. I loved him and we were happy while we were together." The average age of first marriage for women fell from 21.5 to 20.3 in the 1940s while the figure for men showed a fall from 24.3 to 22.7. The percentage of women fifteen years or older who were married rose from 57.5 percent in 1940 to 62.5 percent in 1944, and during the war the birthrate rose from 19.4 to 24.4 per thousand of the population during the war. This reflected the urgency the war brought to human relations, but also the renewal of prosperity.

Although many of these marriages were heat-of-the-moment commitments, the war had a major influence in boosting the family as a key patriotic unit and foundation of American society. Crucial in this process was the powerful emotive use of the family in propaganda: "The man is going off to fight and the only thing that is real and eternal to him is the present moment. The girl he loves becomes the symbol of all life, the life that he is fighting for and expects to come back to. . . . She represents the home that he will forego for the present, the security he will dream of, the children he will hope for."

Again and again the enemy was portrayed in posters and ads as challenging the family. In one ad the Axis powers appear as Halloween vandals who have destroyed a family farm by fire. Behind a tree Uncle Sam stands armed with a rifle representing American industrial power. Soldiers were asked to risk their lives for those they loved and for their mothers—who would be presented with a blue-star flag if they had a son in the army and a gold star if their son was killed. Hollywood showed soldiers fighting for their brides, fiancées, moms, and kids. In *Guadalcanal Diary* (1943), a marine captain lies dying on the beach. As he draws his last breath, he grabs his helmet with his family's photograph inside it. For those without girls at home, Hollywood and the government promoted the great pin-up poster of the actress Betty Grable in a white swimsuit taken from behind and smiling over her shoulder. Grable's picture certainly had an erotic force: she represented American womanhood for whom the GI was risking his life. She was "model, girlfriend, and finally mother." Her marriage to bandleader Harry James and her subsequent motherhood only increased her popularity.

On the home front, the appeal to the family was no less potent. A radio segment, "To the Young," included this piece:

> YOUNG MAN'S VOICE: That's one of the things this war's about.
> YOUNG FEMALE VOICE: About us.
> YOUNG MALE VOICE: About all young people like us. About love and gettin' hitched, and havin' a home and some kids, and breathin' fresh air out in the suburbs . . . about livin' and workin' decent like free people.

Media aimed at women also powerfully stressed the force of the family. William Wyler's Oscar-winning 1942 film *Mrs. Miniver,* with Greer Garson playing a British housewife on the home front, portrayed the courage and tenacity of women during war. Much propaganda urged women to get out and work, but even these appeals were couched in terms of doing one's bit for family and home. Women defense workers were told that they were "fighting for freedom and all that means to women everywhere. You're fighting for a little house of your own, and a husband to meet every night at the door. You're fighting for the right to bring up your children without the shadow of fear."

The home remained women's first priority. *McCall's* magazine in 1943 wrote approvingly of the results of a survey: "very emphatically" the view was that "a woman's place is in the home." Women's employment was always considered a temporary expedient, only for the duration of the war. General Electric announced that women would be glad to go back "to the old housekeeping routine" because their new appliances would make housework much easier. Eureka vacuum cleaners praised women on the assembly line but promised that, once the war was over, "Like you, Mrs. America, Eureka would put aside its uniform and return to the ways of peace . . . building household appliances." An ad for Tangee admitted that wearing lipstick alone was not sufficient to win the war: "But it symbolizes one of the reasons why we are fighting . . . the precious right of women to be feminine and lovely." A handcream manufacturer noted that "Barbara is romantically lovely with her . . . white, flowerlike skin, but she's also TODAY'S American Girl, energetically at work six days a week in a big war plant." Women's magazines urged their readers to keep up their skills as homemakers and consumers as a matter of pride. Experts advised women to develop the talents of nutritionist, decorator, and childrearer. Advertising stressed the rewards to come after the war. The Revere Copper company declared, "Youth has a new world to look forward to. For today's young man and woman can plan as well as dream, can be sure that the homes their parents wished for can become a reality for them. . . . In this war, we are fighting not only against our enemies but for a better way of life for many more of us."

The work of the painter Norman Rockwell especially recognized the link between the family and patriotism and pursued it. Originally published in the *Saturday Evening Post* in 1943, the *Four Freedoms* illustrations were eventually reprinted millions of times. In *Freedom from Fear,* an anxious mother and father, having read in a newspaper of the bombing of London, look on as their children sleep. In *Freedom from Want,* a Thanksgiving family dinner is lovingly portrayed. The aim of these illustrations was to show that Americans were fighting for their families' material benefit. The posters became so popular because they touched a patriotic nerve.

It is scarcely surprising, then, that marriage continued to be central to women's lives in the 1940s, upheld by the economic boom that made it possible for thousands to marry. In 1940 the marriage rate was 105 per thousand, compared to 89.1 in the "normal" years of 1925 to 1929. Between 1940 and 1943, one million more families were created than might have been expected in more ordinary times.

The movies joined in this renewed emphasis on parenthood and the importance of the family. In the 1941 film *Penny Serenade,* starring Irene Dunne and Cary Grant, a couple marry and look forward to the birth of their child. But Dunne's character, Julie, miscarries when an earthquake occurs. So they adopt a child. But when Grant's character loses his job, they become destitute and in danger of losing the child. Grant pleads to the judge to permit him to keep the baby by making a powerful paean to fatherhood: "Please judge, I'll sell anything I got until I get going again. . . . She'll never go hungry and she'll never be without clothes, not as long as I've got two good hands to help me."

Motherhood too took on new meaning. A brace of movie stars who had previously been featured for their voluptuousness now revealed the joys of pregnancy and motherhood. The actress Maureen O'Hara wrote, "I am waiting for my baby. . . . I am aware of the power [my body] holds. It's a kind of spiritual awareness, a reverence, because within me I feel the gentle movement of another body." Elsewhere Joan Crawford appeared as "another incredibly devoted and capable mother."

In keeping with the cultural message, there occurred a considerable increase in the birthrate. The figure of 18 or 19 per thousand during the depression had been the lowest in history.

But by 1941 the figure had risen to 20.4. And in 1943 it was 22.7. All the same, access to birth control increased. By the early 1940s seven Southern states instituted family planning services in their public health programs. Even Roman Catholics felt able to practice birth control after Pope Pius XI in 1930 sanctioned the rhythm method. The use of condoms also increased. Among African-American women, however, only one in five practiced birth control, compared to 83 to 89 percent of white urban women.

The media and propaganda images that bolstered the family thus carried great potency for Americans at war. But not all propaganda and media affirmed traditional images of domesticity. Female characters in comic adventure strips aimed at soldiers became extremely active, rescuing such beleaguered males as Buck Rogers and Flash Gordon. Wonder Woman hailed from the Amazon utopia of Paradise Island and came with a mission "to save the world from the hatred and wars of men in a man-made world." She represented a new self-reliant woman who was capable of looking after the nation's economy while the men were away. The cartoonist Milton Caniff went one step further in liberating women by creating "Miss Lace," the star of "Male Call." This comic was particularly directed at GIs: "a girl strip, as racy as is permissible . . . designed to appeal specially to the forlorn figure in the fox-hole." Miss Lace appeared wearing very little in a variety of military situations. In one notable story, soldiers spied on her as she sunbathed naked. This cartoon upset and scandalized some religious leaders, but others praised it for "the clever and tasteful way in which you treat the fighting man's frank and animal interest in the opposite sex." War, like depression, could help taboos.

The forces that had been building to undermine Victorian morality combined to gain ground with other regards. The freedoms of urban teenagers continued to grow. Premarital pregnancy, illegitimacy, and venereal disease rates all rose. A minor panic in fact ensued over the growth of "sex delinquency" as "Victory Girls," "Khaki Wackies," and "Free Girls" willingly lined up to service the troops. FBI statistics revealed a 95 percent rise between 1940 and 1944 in women accused of morals violations. By way of comparison, charges for prostitution rose only 17.6 percent. "Wolf Packs," or female youth gangs, appeared. Sexual relations with male gang members was a common initiation. Late in the war, Victory Girls who had been charged with morals violations were required to undergo a counseling program. But they were not expected to be medically tested or held in quarantine. A number of the women detained on morals charges were in fact married women with husbands serving in the military. This seems to confirm the observation of the postwar Kinsey Report of an increase in infidelity among young marrieds during the war.

At the same time Mexican and African-American youth became more assertive of their own identity, developing many of the characteristics of a subculture. Teenage boys, especially in poorer areas, dressed in zoot suits—loosely cut coats with padded shoulders and pants that flared down to the knee and then tapered off to the ankle. To many observers this style seemed unnecessarily aggressive in its self-conscious rejection of the staid Victorian suit. But racial fears of an uncontrolled sexuality were unleashed as girls joined the Zoot Suiters with their own gangs, the Slick Chicks and the Black Widows. The latter group wore black zoot-suit jackets, black shirts, and black fishnet stockings, challenging expectations of respectable white female behavior.

Girls also became bobby soxers who swooned over Frank Sinatra while they read such new magazines as *Glamour* and *Mademoiselle* that were directed at them. By the 1940s the idea of youth as a distinctive time of life had become well established. "Teen culture" grew stronger as wartime jobs permitted young people to earn a little spare cash for magazines, records, and clothes.

Finally, the war brought fresh freedoms to gays. The military enabled gay men, previously isolated in small towns, to meet one another and create their own homoerotic world. The military, as ever, tried to weed out homosexuals or "sexual psychopaths," as they were called. On induction, all new recruits were asked about their sexual preferences. Few men were likely to admit to homosexuality, even if they did not wish to fight. A large number of gay men thus entered the army. But here was unparalleled opportunity for contact with other men. One veteran described how the army managed a "gay ambience" during the war. According to Alan Berube's standard study, "Servicemen openly cruised each other in the anonymity of crowded bus and train stations, city parks, restrooms and YMCAs, beaches and streets. They doubled up in hotel beds, slept on the floor in movie theaters, and went home with strangers when there was nowhere else to sleep." The networks and links among gay men that were established during the war laid the foundation of a nationwide and visible gay minority that was to be a far cry from the isolated, underworld homoerotic culture of Victorian times.

Lesbians too found each other. When Mildred from upstate New York went off harvesting with the Land Army and saw two women kissing, she became concerned. On being told they were lesbians, she realized, "For the first time, I had a name for myself." Juanita Loveless recalls a greater tolerance of sexual diversity: "We accepted people then."

The war thus helped promote continued movement away from traditional morality by providing multifarious opportunities for the practice of sexualities, both heterosexual and homosexual, that challenged the norm. The question that remained was whether, once the war was won and millions of Americans returned to civilian life, they would be willing to return to resume married life and set up the safe and secure families that so much propaganda had insisted they had been fighting for. Or would the revolt against Victorian morality gather force?

5

A Return to Victorianism?

AMERICANS after World War II had a great deal to be proud of. They had come out of the war relatively unscathed. After a period of caution, when the American economy pulled painlessly out of a brief downturn in 1947–1948, confidence returned. The United States then invested billions of dollars of Marshall Plan aid in the Western European economies. Belief in the American way seemed justified. And as the benefits of trade with the reviving European economies filtered across the Atlantic to create a series of booms in the 1950s, most Americans understood that here was a mid-century "American High" to be savored.

Americans now sought, above all, stability in their personal lives with which to enjoy the fruits of their labors. Having come through the traumas of depression and war, they felt they deserved the good life. Three sets of extraordinary statistics show that Americans were as successful in their personal lives as they were economically and on the international stage. First of all, women were marrying younger. In 1940 they had on average married at 21.5 years. But by 1956 the average age of marriage was 20.1.

Second, the birthrate rose. In 1940 there had been only 19.4 births per thousand. By the 1957 peak, the figure was 25.3. Women who came of age during the 1930s bore an average of 2.4 children; those who came of age in the 1950s were to bear

an average of 3.2. Women were having more children, and
though these children—the baby boomers—were eventually
to challenge Victorian morality anew, the increase in births
was for the time being an affirmation of traditional values: the
downward spiral of the birthrate had been arrested.

Third, and perhaps most curiously, the divorce rate, after
rising for a generation, fell. In 1946, following the inevitable
disruptions to relationships of the war, it peaked at 4.3 per
thousand married. But by 1958 it had fallen to 2.1 per thousand. This was an amazing reversal. No wonder that in the
1940s and 1950s a massive amount of literature appeared that
celebrated the American family, with parenthood at its core.
The writer Landon Jones called it "a Progressive ethic," a "re-
productive consensus": nonprocreative sexuality was unacceptable as Americans played hard at making babies.

The strongest sign of this attitude was a revitalized cult of
domesticity. Now both women and men were included. Domesticity became a key theme of Hollywood films. Movie stars
were photographed not coming out of the divorce courts but
together as man and wife. Claudette Colbert appeared with
her husband above the caption, "Step over this charming
threshold and meet—not a star and her husband—but a doctor and his wife." Colbert wrote that it was hard to "take care
of three children and be a bundle of charm at day's end . . .
that is what man has expected of a wife since the world
began." She advised women to try to be "gay and interesting
when he is at home." Joan Crawford turned up in a photograph cleaning the floor, wearing an apron; this, the caption
read, was the "real" Joan Crawford, taking care of her domestic duties when not acting. In 1946 Jane Wyman and Ronald
Reagan were featured in *Photoplay* magazine having a
friendly lovers' tiff. "Go away. You bother me," said Jane, who
then continued with remarkable foresight: "Go get the world
straightened out and then maybe I'll talk to you." As the cap-

tion writer noted, with even more prescience, "Rest assured, if it were up to Ronnie, he's the one man who could do it!"

The stress on motherhood as the fulfillment of women's sexuality continued. Marynia Farnham and Ferdinand Lundberg's *Modern Woman: The Lost Sex* (1947) was typical, though it was not as widely distributed as has often been claimed. By way of contrast, from its publication in 1946 right up to the present, Dr. Benjamin Spock's *Baby and Childcare* was a huge success. It insisted on the centrality of the mother to the bringing up of a child. Women needed to be with their children during their first five years of life, Spock maintained. Any psychological difficulties or juvenile delinquency that might afflict the child were the fault of the mother. Yet Spock's book, for all its blaming of women, helped cement the revived idea of family and traditional values.

For a change, fathers too featured as major players in the raising of children. The dim and distant figure of the Victorian patriarch was now replaced by the image of the suburban father. *Life* in 1954 announced "the domestication of the American male." Fathers were asked "Are you a Dad or a dud?" For many Americans, the cult of "togetherness" and of parenthood came together when life imitated art on the television set in *I Love Lucy*. Lucy and her husband Ricky Ricardo proclaimed the birth of both their TV and real-life child at the same time. The nation swooned at this very public display of happy families.

Parenthood indeed took on a whole new dimension in these years. For Louisa Randall Church, writing in 1946, parents in the era of the atomic age assumed "added responsibilities of deep and profound significance. Surely, in all history, the parents of the world were never so challenged!" For children were now "a defense—an impregnable bulwark against the fears and anxieties of the era." The historian Elaine Tyler May argues there was even more responsibility in the parental role:

"For men who were frustrated at work, for women who were bored at home, and for both who were dissatisfied with the unfulfilled promises of sexual excitement, children might fill the void." Much evidence like this suggests that the "happy family" image may well have masked burdens and demands.

The potent new medium of television spread domesticity and family values. Fatherhood on TV appeared central to men's identity. Yet this was not the breadwinner ethic of men in the real world. TV fathers such as Ward Cleaver and Ozzie Nelson defined their manhood through the resolution of their children's problems. *Leave It to Beaver, Father Knows Best, Ozzie and Harriet,* and *I Love Lucy* became the clichés of what the 1950s American family was like. These TV shows revealed comfortable suburban families where the children's minor misdemeanors were sorted out by kindly parents and grandparents. But TV advertising also encouraged this idea. A 1956 ad for Chevrolet argued strongly for the two-car family: "Going our separate ways, we've never been so close. The family with two cars gets twice as many chores completed, so there's more leisure to enjoy TOGETHER." The world of TV offered stability through clear roles: Jim Anderson of *Father Knows Best* and Ward Cleaver left for work each morning. Mothers nurtured their families with the aid of the modern conveniences in their homes. Only Ricky Nelson's singing threatened the idyll.

Togetherness, then, was the secret to success. Scenes of father, mom, and the children in the bliss of domesticity were everywhere in 1950s advertising and magazine articles. Everybody got married. The *Women's Guide to Better Living* advised, "Whether you are a man or a woman, the family is the unit to which you most genuinely belong. . . . The family is the center of your living. If it isn't, you've gone far astray." Paul Landis, a marriage counselor, proclaimed that "Marriage is the natural state of adults." Wedded bliss was the way to fulfill President Dwight D. Eisenhower's dictum to "be happy every day." As if to confirm this, media showed couples in love embracing in the gardens of their homes in the suburbs. Just as Victorians had seen the triumph of American industrial growth vindicated in the success of their families, so in the 1950s the success of the American economy seemed to be confirmed by millions of happy families in suburbias throughout the country.

Happy though these families usually were, family stability suited the American government very well in the fight against communism. At the end of the decade, Vice President Richard Nixon, himself a doting and loving father and husband, went to the American Exhibition in Moscow. There he showed off to the Russians all the modern conveniences that made the American housewife's task so easy. Nixon and the model kitchen displayed at the exhibition particularly irritated the bullying Nikita Khrushchev, the Soviet premier. In the cold war fight against communism, the American family was a major bulwark against the encroachment of the evils of the Russian system.

In recent years this positive view of the American family in the 1950s has been challenged by the perspective of Betty Friedan's classic 1963 polemic *The Feminine Mystique*. Friedan's method of subverting family values was to claim her own frustrations with an unhappy marriage and the irritations of her Smith College classmates as the experience of all American women. The resulting work was explosive because, clearly, many American women saw elements of their own lives in Friedan's descriptions. With method and craft, Friedan took a hammer to the American family. She notoriously described the home as a "comfortable concentration camp" in which women's every career aspiration was stifled and thwarted. Women who were afflicted by this "problem that has no name" felt stunted, trapped in a "feminine mystique." While men revered and praised them, they simultaneously were denied their highest needs and aspirations. Friedan presented a powerful indictment of the consequences for women of the emphasis on family over career.

Friedan created a myth not only about her own life but also about what the 1950s were really like. A privileged woman with an Ivy League education, between 1947 and 1962 she had—like a large and growing percentage of American women—pursued a career, marriage, and motherhood. She had worked as a successful labor journalist and propagandist for the most tightly controlled Communist-influenced union, which she took care to conceal for fear it would expose the left-wing agenda underlying her book. And her attack ignored the fact that women's work was not discouraged in the 1950s. Magazines may well have gloried in togetherness and the joys of marriage and motherhood, but they also encouraged women to pursue careers. Friedan herself had written articles such as "Why I Went Back to Work," which seemingly would have been impossible in the world she imagined in *The Feminine Mystique*. But our image of the fifties has been clouded by this book not least because historians have taken to examining approving letters written to Friedan on its publication as evidence for the truth of what it contains. They have, however, ignored the objecting letters she received when she published an article called "The Fraud of Feminism" in *McCall's* magazine. A great many women wrote in to defend marriage and the family. One declared, "I am a proud and fulfilled wife." Another insisted, "I will not be a sheep following the rest of the herd because I have certain ideas and ideals." The defenders of domesticity were also vocal in these years.

Yet there were other undercurrents of rebellion. After the war the sexual ferment continued, portrayed in the works of the sexologist Alfred Kinsey. In two scholarly books, *Sexual Behavior in the Human Male* (1948) and *Sexual Behavior in the*

Human Female (1953), this internationally renowned expert on the gall wasp changed the American public's perception of sexual morality and behavior. Kinsey's findings, the results of interviews over a number of years with a wide cross section of Americans, caused a sensation. The volume on men attracted so much attention because of its revelations about homosexual behavior and especially its claims that 37 percent of men had had sex to orgasm with another man at some time from adolescence onward. Between ages sixteen and fifty-five, 10 percent of males had had exclusively homosexual intercourse for a period of at least three years. Although the gay movement was later to take this figure as a rallying cry, in fact Kinsey's report is clear that only 4 percent of males were "exclusively homosexual" over their entire lifetime. Nevertheless, this information was a bombshell. Kinsey devised a continuum according to which sexual behavior was placed on a scale of zero to six. Zero meant exclusively homosexual; six exclusively heterosexual. The implication that homosexuality and bisexuality were as normal as heterosexuality caused more furor. Kinsey's contention that only half of male orgasms occurred in marriage also stirred up moralists. When did the rest occur? a nation wondered—and Victorian innocence crumbled further.

Kinsey's study of American females in 1953 further subverted what remained of Victorian morality. Kinsey found that 26 percent of women had experienced intercourse outside of marriage, 80 percent had petted before marriage, and half had had premarital intercourse, usually with the partner they were going to marry. But few women were promiscuous. Again these figures revealed the extent to which Americans routinely broke away from traditional and religious ideals.

Kinsey revolutionized the study of sex because he approached it as a "passionate reformer" who believed that "sex was good." Previous sex studies had assumed that they served a moral purpose—indeed, they aimed to support Victorian morality. By way of contrast, Kinsey reveled in an ethic of sexual liberation while hiding behind the veneer of scientific respectability and rationality that his status as a university professor gave him. As his biographer James H. Jones notes, he saw "civilization as the enemy of sex," and he appeared as a man determined to justify his own homosexual feelings by exposing how common were sexualities that had been considered deviant. Thus Kinsey, writing in the forties and fifties, heralded the so-called sexual revolution of the sixties and seventies.

He repeatedly declared throughout his work the extent to which his study undermined earlier assumptions. He insisted, for example, that intercourse outside of marriage did not weaken marital stability. And on homosexuality he directly challenged the view that same-sex relations are "rare and therefore abnormal or unnatural, or that they constitute within themselves evidence of neurosis or even psychosis." He went on to say that "the capacity of an individual to respond erotically to any sort of stimulus, whether it is provided by another person of the same or of the opposite sex, is basic to the species." As a biologist/zoologist, Kinsey saw sex in terms of "outlet." He insisted that "Biologically, there is no form of outlet that I will admit as abnormal." Kinsey thus removed all moral content from the study of sex. This was recognized early on by Kinsey's fellow Indiana University professor Thurman Rice, who believed in the tradition that sex research was a subject of moral, not scientific, inquiry. Rice, a defender of traditional morality, became the bane of Kinsey's life and challenged him at every turn. More practically, he helped ensure that many of the sources of Kinsey's funding were cut. Yet Kinsey's importance cannot be denied. He laid the groundwork for far more radical and revolutionary figures in the 1960s and 1970s.

Some observers suggest that it was men who first revolted against the demands of marriage. Most men in the 1950s got married and stayed married. But they did fantasize. This need was appreciated by Hugh Hefner, whose *Playboy* magazine took the values of this male yearning right into the mainstream American home, making him a multi-millionaire in the process. *Playboy*'s first issue, with its famous Marilyn Monroe nude, sold fifty thousand copies in 1953, outselling *Esquire,* the previous leader in men's magazines. Hefner's genius was not so much, as one wag indicated, "to link sex with upward mobility" as to appreciate that "men liked looking at women's breasts, and lots of them, the bigger the better." Hefner realized that men would be most interested in ogling the mammaries of two kinds of women—movie stars and "girls next door." The latter were easy to find, and relatively inexpensive models. Hefner persuaded his subscription manager, Charlaine Karalus to strip for *Playboy* under the pseudonym of Janet Pilgrim. She was an enormous success and became a celebrity, appearing as a "centerfold" in July 1955, December 1955, and October 1956. A *Playboy* salesman found a client's secretary, Jacquelyn Prescott, to pose for the magazine, both at work, clothed, and away from work—in the nude. These pin-ups were extremely popular, suggesting to men that the girl next door was also interested in sex. But the magazine also gave men unrealistic expectations of what they might encounter in real life. How many wives could match up?

Few wives could compare anyway with the movie stars who were increasingly featured in the pages of the magazine. Marilyn Monroe's famous nude in the first issue coincided with her first real taste of stardom in *Gentlemen Prefer Blondes* (1953). Others soon followed suit. Jayne Mansfield, a Monroe imitator, first appeared in February 1955, while the daring studies of Anita Ekberg published in 1956 encouraged *Time* to observe that "*Esquire* cannot keep abreast of *Playboy*" because in *Esquire* Ekberg had "a few clothes on." Kim Novak's career gained greatly by her appearance in a 1959 issue of *Playboy*. But the magazine was most effective in advancing the reputations of foreign actresses. Three features on Brigitte Bardot appeared, promoting her husband director Roger Vadim's film *And God Created Woman* (1956), and she established herself in the United States as "Europe's favorite sex kitten." A November 1957 still from an Italian Sophia Loren film introduced that actress. In *Playboy* ordinary American men could see extraordinary women naked; this was fun compared with their staid home lives.

Hefner, in an effort to draw in mainstream advertisers, tried hard to determine who *Playboy*'s actual audience was. "What is a Playboy?" asked a long-running subscription caption. "Is he simply a wastrel, a ne'er do well, a fashionable bum?" No, "far from it: he can be a sharp-minded business executive, a worker in the arts, a university professor, an architect or engineer." Hefner went on: "He can be many things, providing he possesses a certain point of view. He must see life not as a vale of tears, but as a happy time: he must take joy in his work, without regarding it as the end and all of living." A Playboy must, most importantly, be a man who "without acquiring the stigma of the voluptuary or dilettante—can live life to the hilt." A series of advertisements that asked "What sort of man reads *Playboy*?" pictured *Playboy* readers as businessmen, beachboys, skiers, and car drivers. In other words, every American man could be a Playboy. Yet most *Playboy* readers were married. They had jobs. They were fathers. They had children. *Playboy* man, however, still could have a "point of view." He must enjoy "mixing up cocktails and an hors d'oeuvre or putting a little mood music on the phonograph and inviting in a female acquaintance for a quiet discussion on Picasso, Nietzsche, jazz, sex." As the magazine's first editorial indicated, "We want to make it clear from the very start, we aren't a 'family magazine.' If you're somebody's sister, wife or mother-in-law and picked us up by mistake, please pass us along to the man in your life and get back to your *Ladies' Home Companion.*" With *Playboy,* ordinary married men could fantasize about being unmarried, and those who were not married could fantasize about avoiding getting married! All the same, this was just a relatively mild revolt against family values, and indeed it could be argued that the vicarious gratification of fantasy served as a safety valve for marriage. Still, Hefner was in the tradition of the *Police Gazette* and the Macfadden journals. He knew that sex sold, and in a climate of strong sexual control he became a millionaire. And the portrayal of women as sexual objects in the magazine represented a far stronger assault on older values of female purity.

No one more embraced the idea of women as sex object than Marilyn Monroe. Monroe's life story and her tragedy will be familiar to readers. But she came along at exactly the right time: just as a male fantasy world outside marriage and the family was emerging in American culture. Monroe was the victim of the millions of fantasies about her. She needed those fantasies just as the excessive demands they placed on her finally destroyed her. Monroe's role in the revolt against Victorian sexual morality is more complex. She was no Mae West. Mae West was brazen, albeit with a keen business mind and sense of humor. Although highly sexual and sexually attractive, Monroe combined some of the chief characteristics of Victorianism: she was submissive and passive. She embodied the extent to which 1950s Americans, even in their advocacy of family values, embraced openly a highly sexually charged society.

Although most women were satisfied with marriage in the 1950s, they too felt undercurrents of revolt. Women's dissatisfaction can be traced to the extreme sexualization of marriage that seemed to gain renewed intensity in the decade. Some

argue that this resulted from the continuing taboo against premarital sexual intercourse, which in turn created an unprecedented premium on sex in marriage itself. What is clear is that
1950s Americans seemed to see successful sex in marriage as a
panacea. They carried the cult of the mutual orgasm onward
and upward and beyond. Children would be made unhappy if
their parents suffered from sexual frustration; a child expert
declared: "the matter . . . of sexual adjustment between the
parents was 'found to be related to children's difficulties and
maladjustments to a very important degree.'" An array of
similar psychologists and educators celebrated sexuality in
marriage. And Van de Velde's marriage manual's popularity
continued: the family had to "fulfill virtually all its members'
personal needs through an energized and expressive personal
life."

Sexual attraction became the main rationale for marriage.
One writer declared that "60 percent profound affection and
respect [and] 40 percent intense sex attraction" made for a
good marriage. Should one attain this, "you can be fairly sure
that you'll get the happy, fantastic fairytale result." Men and
women really believed all this. Surveys revealed that "physical
attraction" or "sexual desire" was a major reason for marriage.
One woman wrote that her fiancé was "easy on the eye." For
men, this need to be attractive led to enough difficulties; they
had distinctive standards to live up to. But for women it was
even worse. Magazines, advertisements, and, perhaps most
stress-creating, movie stars defined an allure that women had
to match. This allure was, of course, a major component of attracting a man and a major factor in keeping him with you.

By the 1950s many women, comfortable and privileged in a
land of abundance, demanded sexual satisfaction as a right.
And marriage was the only place to find it. One woman has
described how "sex was lousy at first. Well, we were both virgins, what do you expect? Neither of us knew a thing about

what to do. I didn't have my first orgasm until we'd been married for several years. It was an accident." Some women were prepared to look elsewhere for gratification, as men had always done. A woman called Dorothy wrote that "I was 32 or 33 and I guess I was at the height of my sexuality. The problem was we just weren't having sex very much. We could go for a year without having sex. . . . I had to leave. . . . I had an affair . . . mainly to check out the idea that it wasn't my fault." Betty Friedan interviewed a thirty-year-old mother of five who told her that "she was thinking of going away, to Mexico perhaps, to live with a man with whom she was having an affair." "What about the children?" asked Friedan. "Vaguely, she guessed she would take them along—he wouldn't mind." This woman remembered how she had felt when she married her husband at eighteen—"I felt so happy I wanted to die." Victorian women had enjoyed sex and expected to enjoy sex. But they had grinned and borne it when things did not go well: the institution of marriage had had so many other purposes that it could survive the breakdown of sexual felicity. By the 1950s the other functions of marriage had become less important than sexual gratification and satisfaction.

On the path to marriage, dating, the cause of such concern in the 1920s and 1930s, now scarcely raised an eyebrow. After World War II the dating system became part of the postwar high school culture of soda pop, Chevrolets, and diners. Young people found that more money gave them greater leeway as consumers. A poll of young Minnesotans in 1946 asked at what age they should begin to date. It found that only 1 percent believed young people should not date at all. More than three-quarters of boys and girls thought they should start dating before the age of seventeen. Even more striking, dating no longer caused generational conflict. Parents who had themselves dated saw no harm in it. A comparison of polls examining relationships with parents showed that the number of dates, or quarrels over where to go on a date, had brought half of girls into conflict with their parents in 1939; but in 1956 this was a problem for only one in nine.

What did shock in the 1950s was the appearance of a new phase of courtship in between dating and engagement—"going steady." The Roper organization in 1955 and 1963 asked parents whether they thought that high school boys and girls ought to go steady. Two-thirds of parents thought not. To parents in the 1950s, going steady was incomprehensible. As an article in *Parents* magazine confirmed, "Going steady doesn't mean anything like being engaged. . . . Where we read marital implications, they read popularity and security." This showed how much adolescents looked to their peers for appropriate courtship behavior, experiencing what the rock writer Jon Savage has called "an acute sense of difference from the adult world."

Social success in high school now depended on having a steady boyfriend or girlfriend. But this seemingly harmless phase had the power to shock because those going steady could pet. As the sociologist Ira Reiss explained it, "High school couples who are going steady . . . feel it is proper to engage in heavy petting . . . the justification being that they are in love or at least extremely fond of each other." Reiss in 1960 dubbed the new moral code "permissiveness with affection," and it became the byword among sociologists for American courtship through to 1970 and beyond. Going steady broke further away from the Victorian system because the courtship period was extended to a series of relationships of varying intensity but of far greater closeness than had been allowable before, outside of engagement. "Permissiveness with affection" acknowledged that boys and girls could become close with many different people before they settled down. As the oral historian Brett Harvey has put it: "Going steady was actually a form of teenage rebellion in the fifties. Parents, educators, and

teen advice-givers inveighed against the practice, suspect-
ing—correctly—that it provided sanctions for necking and
petting." Now the mass of young Americans could practice
the "varietism" that the Greenwich Village bohemians had
advocated earlier in the century. In other words, going steady
was just one more step toward the permissive society, even
though it involved a degree of commitment.

In the 1920s young people had argued about sexual boundaries; but their arguments seem innocent by comparison with
what occurred in the 1950s. Polls and interviews give us snap-
shots of how young people thought at different times. In a
1949 survey of high schoolers, 10 percent of boys thought it
wrong to "pet" or "neck" when they were on dates as against
26 percent of girls. But the numbers of those who thought "intimate petting should be delayed until after marriage" actually
grew a bit. Thus while American teenagers in the 1950s tolerated sexual experimentation, there were limits. Surveys
showed clearly that premarital intercourse was still frowned
upon even if widely practiced among engaged couples. Homosexuality remained generally taboo. But petting was acceptable as long as it took place in the context of affection and
intimacy.

This was all pretty vague. Young people were left with a
great deal of leeway and a vast amount for them to argue
about. And argue they did. An oral history records one
woman's recollections: "His left hand has insinuated itself
under her coat under her sweater, and rests firmly on the
stitched cotton point of her right-bra cup. Her right hand
rests, ever-so-lightly, on his crotch, ready at a moment's notice
to fly up and block his left hand should it venture under her
bra, or attempt a descent to the waistband of her skirt. In the
game of sex as we played it in the fifties, he is on 'second base.'
If he 'gets lucky' she will 'go all the way' and he will have
'scored.' "

The major dilemma young people faced was how far to go, and the responsibility for this decision rested squarely with the woman. As one woman described a situation: "In my junior year, this boy, Terry, took a shine to me. He used to drive out to the farm to take me out and we would have these long struggles in the car. I wasn't even that attracted to him—I was just so grateful to have somebody interested in me. So in these struggles I wasn't at war with my own impulses so much as just keeping him at arm's length for all I was worth." Another woman talks of how her boyfriend, Charlie, respected her and regarded her as the "kind of girl I want to marry" because she constantly resisted him. "We had terrible fights in the car, Charlie and I. The thing was, though, even though we acted out this struggle—he'd push push push, I'd say stop stop stop—we both knew the rules." For another woman, her dating of a campus star led to a terrific row: "Well, one night it got way out of hand and I just let myself go and all of a sudden I realized he wasn't going to stop and at the same moment he was in. Well, he pulled out right away, I mean we kind of wrenched away from each other. Then we proceeded to have this terrible fight." She pleaded, "I can't believe it—you were going to do it," while he accused her—"You *let* me! Why didn't you stop me?" In a world where the double standard remained powerful, girls faced the possibility that they might be considered "cheap" and hence lose value on the market.

Bitterness created by the lack of clarity over limits led to the creation in the 1950s of codes of behavior by responsible youth and parents in several high schools. They established clearly what young people had to do in relation to their parents, and also clarified to some extent how the young should behave at parties and on dates. But the codes were too squeamish to discuss sexual matters directly, and as a result they had little impact.

In this context, "going all the way" became a symbol of rebellion for many of the 1950s young. One woman wrote of how she took one look at a certain man and "knew *he* was going to get it." She continues: "I don't know where I got the idea that I shouldn't do it, that it wasn't nice to do it. It wasn't from my parents. We were bohemians! I knew I was an outlaw and part of me didn't want to be." She went away with her man: "We got in my bed and 'did it.' All the time we were doing it, I kept thinking over and over, 'This is it, this is it, this is what it is.'" Another woman has written of how she was very conventional, went steady all the way through college, but then met a man at work with whom she began a passionate affair: "I moved in with this man for a week. Can you imagine?" She continues, "But this was the first time I had ever really dared to do anything that I knew was wrong. I was compelled, I was excited. I couldn't help myself. But in a way I was glad I did it, because it was ME doing it! I wasn't doing it to please anyone, for the first time in my life."

But the 1950s had darker, bleaker undercurrents that came to the surface in the juvenile delinquency scare. By the early fifties Hollywood began to relax its strict censorship code. Audiences were dwindling, and studios realized that they needed to appeal to teenagers; so the code was eased gently. The resulting genre of teen films explored the teenage experience and in the process created stars who revised standards of sexual morality and expanded sexual boundaries. The first and greatest to emerge from this category (which he soon transcended) was Marlon Brando. The product of Irish rough culture, Brando had made his reputation in 1946 in a tight and torn T-shirt in *A Streetcar Named Desire* on Broadway. In Stanley Kramer's *The Wild One* (1953), Brando played the part of the archetypal sexual rebel. Mean and moody and sexually ambiguous, this bike rider seems to have come straight out of the underworld to terrorize a small town. He is only fleetingly tender with his lover whom he soon deserts, leaving her to face the small town he has upset. The 1950s Brando, in a series of other films, most notably *On the Waterfront* (1954), became the epitome of a new kind of male "cool." He brought lower-class sexual attractiveness and rough-tough maleness to the American middle class. If Fairbanks had been genuinely middle class and Valentino safely exotic, Brando was definitely American and working class without any trace of regard for middle-class mores and niceties. The 1951 film of *A Streetcar Named Desire* especially caused a huge fuss with the censors at the time. The Production Code Administration objected strongly to its depiction of "homosexuality, nymphomania, and rape." Joe Breen, still censoring into the 1950s, wrote that "Homosexuality is not mentionable in the American cinema." But the director Elia Kazan stood firm on the rape scene which he regarded as "the heart of the play."

James Dean, even more than Brando, emerged as an icon of the youth culture. At twenty-four, in 1955, he played an adolescent in *Rebel Without a Cause*, the most important of a cycle of juvenile delinquency films. Dean slouches and preens as the hero rebelling against his parents, while displaying an androgynous kind of masculinity; his mannered performance confirmed his own immature sexuality. The message of the film was that all adults were hopelessly unaware of the problems of youth and that salvation lay in teenagers who could go beyond the limitations of the middle-class family. Dean's family appears maladjusted, his mother dominating his weak father, while the teenagers protest the meaninglessness of their parents' relationships while seeking fresh ways to love. Sadly, Dean's potential was never realized as he died in a car accident shortly after the film was released. And his "live fast, die young" ethos as well as his sexual persona soon diffused into rock culture, where it not only influenced Elvis but was taken all too literally by a string of rock stars from Jim Morrison to Kurt Cobain.

The 1955 film *Blackboard Jungle* not only continued the juvenile delinquency theme but also heralded the music of youthful rebellion: rock 'n' roll. Bill Haley and the Comets' *Rock Around the Clock* (1955) became a teen anthem with its rapid rhythm and stirring lyrics. The film proclaimed its moralistic concern with youth's problems in an opening statement: "Today we are concerned with juvenile delinquency— its causes and its effects. We are especially concerned when this delinquency boils over into our schools...." But the movie actually provoked the very delinquency it claimed to be countering. The English teacher, the main adult character, was able to get through to his students, but it was clear he could do this only because he listened to them and sought answers from them. The overall impression of the film, however, is of violence, disrespect for authority, and a rock music whose sheer exuberance and energy seemed to reject all compromise with the adult world.

From the mid-fifties, rock 'n' roll's black and white pioneers caused a cultural revolution among the young through the music's pulsating beat, sensuality, and encouragement of free emotional expression. Parents and authorities loathed it, but the young rapidly embraced the music of rock's pioneers: Chuck Berry, Little Richard, Fats Domino, Carl Perkins, Bo Diddley, Buddy Holly, and the Everly Brothers.

The artist who made the greatest impact was Elvis Presley, who between 1956 and 1960 charted fifteen No. 1 hits and twenty-three top-ten hits. In 1956 he appeared on the scene as a strikingly handsome young man who, outrageously, sang like a black man and moved his body uninhibitedly. As the London *Times* put it, his moves "suggested the fundamental urge." Jack O'Brien of the *New York Journal-American* was not so polite: "Elvis Presley wriggled and wriggled with such abdominal gyrations that burlesque bombshell Georgie Southern really deserves equal time to reply in gyrating kind...."

He can't sing a lick, makes up for vocal shortcomings with the weirdest and plainly planned suggestive animation short of an aborigine's mating dance." Here was "Pelvis Presley" with the "Hootchy Cootchy" mannerisms. Never had a white man been so "all shook up." This song, one of his biggest hits from 1957, epitomized the sheer link to life and passion that lay in the music. Presley declares his love and physical desire with such intense vibrancy that it is not only he who is shaken up; metaphorically, the exuberance and excitement of the song shakes up the bland respectability of adult culture.

A decent, well-brought-up young man who famously loved his mama, Presley pleaded innocent. In interviews he said he could not help but move as he did when he heard the beat: "I jump around because it's the way that I feel." Television tried hard to tame him. When he appeared on the Ed Sullivan Show he could only be shown from the waist up. Yet still he scandalized moralizers. The *New York Times* wrote that "When Presley executes his bumps and grinds, it must be remembered by the Columbia Broadcasting System that even the twelve year old's curiosity may be over-stimulated." Evangelist Billy Graham, admitting that he had not seen Presley, nevertheless wrote, "From what I've heard, I'm not so sure that I'd want my children to see him."

The moralizers were correct to be so concerned. Presley's importance lay not just in that he pioneered the creation of this music of youthful sexual rebellion, but that he brought the black underworld sexuality he had learned growing up in Tupelo, Mississippi, to America's youth. Presley is therefore one of the most influential figures of all in the revolt against Victorian sexual morality. He made music that was thrilling and seemingly dangerous. Here was a male sexuality that, influenced by Dean's and Brando's personae, completely undercut earlier notions of respectability. By comparison, Frank Sinatra, a scandal in his time, seemed dull, old, and insipid. The vast increase in record sales that Presley spearheaded, the host of imitators who sprang up in his wake, and the remarkable staying power in his work and his popularity have assured his stature as a legend. For behind his Southern innocence and politeness and charm, Presley was quite untamable. Until the Beatles came along he led the pack, mostly due to the sheer force of his talent and personality. He was a genius. Yet rock 'n' roll arose at a particular moment, when record companies realized that a growing youth market was receptive to a kind of music strongly African-American in origin, even if largely performed by white stars. Concerns about traditional morality were swept aside as the bottom line grew larger: between 1955 and 1959 record sales quadrupled.

Presley served in the army between 1958 and 1960, which reduced the impact of rock. He continued to evoke the passionate sexuality of the young when he returned to civilian life in 1960 with songs as vital as "(Marie's the Name of) His Latest Flame" and "Little Sister." But other figures also were popular and influential in spreading the erotic exuberance of rock. Writes one critic: "From Fats Domino's 1956 'Blueberry Hill' and the Big Bopper's 1958 'Chantilly Lace' to the Everly Brothers' 1957 'Wake Up Little Susie' and Roy Orbison's 1960 'Only the Lonely,' rock 'n' roll persisted in its loud presentations of the thrills, sexuality, vibrancy, and despairing aloneness of America's youth."

Songs like Jerry Lee Lewis's 1957 "Whole Lotta Shakin' Goin' On" and "Great Balls of Fire," with their shouting, moaning, and the use of slang and innuendo (in Little Richard's 1956 "Tutti Frutti"), reflected in song the young's alienation from the coldness of their parents' generation. Jerry Lee Lewis virtually begs for love and sex: "Shake it, baby, shake it/ A whole lotta shakin' goin' on," or yelps with delight: "Goodness, gracious, great balls of fire!"

Such music also provoked a vehement reaction from authority in a country where traditional morality had made such a comeback. Newspapers demanded, "Does rock 'n' roll cause delinquency?" The Reverend Jimmy Snow railed at rock's beat that contained "evil feeling." Other critics claimed rock was "Communist ideology." In the South, racists feared it was spreading black values. The New Jersey Commission for Public Safety in 1958 banned rock shows: "We find that these programs are not for the good of the community. . . ."

All the same, many conservative artists dominated the charts in the 1950s. Pat Boone, though he made a hilariously clinical version of "Tutti Frutti," was generally Mr. Clean. His sugary songs such as "April Love" and "Love Letters in the Sand" rivaled only Elvis Presley commercially. And a traditional Tin Pan Alley star like Paul Anka could emerge in the late fifties to underscore the dominance in the business of conservative values. Too, the 1950s were probably Frank Sinatra's greatest years, the basis of his formidable reputation. But by now he appealed to a mature audience. With all these qualifications, rock nonetheless represented the cutting edge of a new and far-reaching revolt against traditional values, a revolt that would reach its peak in the mid-1960s.

From the bohemian enclaves of New York and San Francisco came another strand of sexual revolt: the beatniks, who in the fifties pioneered the hippy subculture of the sixties. The beatniks spawned the Beat writers who in recent years have become romantic figures to be looked up to as guides on how to live life. Allen Ginsberg, by the time of his death, was a respected figure in the American mainstream, so much so that one obituary described him as nothing less than "one of the great figures of the twentieth century." Such lavish praise was also given to William Burroughs when he died. Jack Kerouac, similarly, has long been seen as a sexy guy in the mold of James Dean, an author whose *On the Road* (1957) is a kind of bible for some Americans.

Much of the appeal of Kerouac's *On the Road* was surely its extraordinarily explicit language. This tale of how Sal Paradise and Dean Moriarty drive around America in the 1940s is both homophobic and sexist. There are numerous slighting references to "fags" and "queers," and the women in the book —who appear as conquests in every town—appear as vague stereotypes and as sex objects. Dean "didn't care one way or the other . . . so long's I can get that lil ole gal with that lil sumpin down there tween her legs, boy" and "so long's we can eat, son!" With his enormous "dangle," Dean knew "all the girls in Denver." At every new town there is a new girl. Sal "made the acquaintance of a girl and we necked all the way to Indianapolis." For Paradise and Moriarty "sex was the one and only holy thing in life."

The morality of *On the Road* mirrored the lived experience of the author and his Beat writer friends. Sal Paradise is Kerouac himself while Dean Moriarty is Neal Cassady. In real life they were lovers, and this is reflected in the last lines of the novel when, despite the endless conquests of women, Paradise writes, "I think of Dean Moriarty, I even think of old Dean Moriarty the father we never found. . . . I think of Dean Moriarty." Yet both Kerouac and Cassady had many heterosexual relationships. By the age of twenty-nine Cassady was married three times. He always had a suitcase ready so that he could leave whenever he wished.

Yet it was not in their advocacy of promiscuous heterosexuality that the Beats were most notable; so much of their outlook had been advocated by the Greenwich Village bohemians. Rather it was their bold advocacy of homosexuality that was most original. For all the homophobic slurs he put into the mouths of his characters in *On the Road,* Kerouac was a "fellow traveler" of gay people—as the critic Catherine Stimpson has described his position—who had affairs with many, including Cassady and Allen Ginsberg. But it was

Ginsberg and Burroughs who were the most homosexual. Ginsberg was a radical homosexual advocate, as indicated in his poem *Howl,* who lived for thirty years with Peter Orlovsky. Burroughs soon fell in love with a man upon the death of his wife. He ended up for a while in Tangiers in a male brothel taking drugs and having affairs with boys while preparing his celebration of gay sex, *Naked Lunch.*

The Beats and their numerous followers advocated gay and straight promiscuity and revolt against marriage. Their success in both recommending and living such a life makes us query the extent to which the 1950s were such a bleak time for homosexuals. While not exactly a golden age for gays, they were very far from the dark ages of popular imagination.

All the same, the McCarthy era at the start of the fifties did represent a time of fear and terror surrounding the topic of homosexuality. When Undersecretary of State John Peurifoy declared that of ninety-one security risks in the State Department, most "were homosexuals," it stirred up a nationwide anti-homosexual hysteria. A Senate subcommittee was formed to study "the employment of homosexuals in government." In 1950 about sixty homosexual federal employees lost their jobs, while in 1953 President Eisenhower issued Executive Order 10405 which delineated that "sexual perversion" was grounds for removal from the federal government. There was also a general upsurge in the prosecution of homosexuals, with an increase in raids on bars. In Florida after 1955 there began a nine-year investigation into the prevalence of homosexuality in education: one hundred teachers eventually lost their jobs. Yet while this must have created a poisonous atmosphere for many homosexuals, most were able to live their lives in peace.

Curiously, and perhaps ironically, the first proper homosexual rights movement, the Mattachine Society, formed in 1950, was originally made up of Communists. Formed by the transplanted Englishman Harry Hay, who was convinced that America was on the verge of fascism, the organization soon grew. In 1952 the ultra-secretive Mattachine successfully defended a member who had been entrapped in a Los Angeles park. This proved a huge spur to the group, which now accepted a wide spectrum of members. By May 1953 it had grown to two thousand people, with a monthly magazine called *One*. Questions about the Communist nature of the leadership led to the resignation of the founders. Yet the organization continued to flourish in its more moderate guise, and chapters appeared throughout the country, focusing on education of the public about homosexuality. The Mattachine soon was under FBI surveillance, its lectures tape-recorded. At Denver in 1959, so confident were the Mattachine that their leaders appeared to the press at a public meeting, only to be raided by the police a few weeks later. But this pattern of harassment was not repeated elsewhere. For although the Mattachine represented a more mainstream acceptance of homosexuality, it was not a subversive group at all. Once the Communist leadership had been removed, the group went out of its way to establish that, apart from their bed preferences, homosexuals were no different from other Americans—in other words, they were good patriotic citizens of the United States.

More important, a homoerotic culture that was in some ways a good deal more daring than the Mattachine was increasingly influencing the mainstream. Gore Vidal is a case in point. His 1948 novel *The City and the Pillar* anticipated many of the arguments of gay liberation. The Vidal stand-in, Paul Sullivan, makes a determined speech in a New Orleans homosexual bar: "[In] America we're sick with fear. . . . We cannot even love. The men cannot love women, cannot love one another, cannot love themselves. . . . No, we must declare ourselves, become known; allow the world to discover this subterranean life of ours which connects kings and farm boys, artists and clerks. Let them see that the important thing is NOT the object of love but the emotion itself, and let them respect anyone, no matter how different he is, if he attempts to share himself with another. . . ." A similarly courageous novel was James Baldwin's *Giovanni's Room,* published in 1956. This story of an American in Paris who falls in love with an Italian waiter was bold for the time and could only be published in the United States after it had been published in Britain. The playwright Tennessee Williams was not as openly daring in his plays, but one could easily detect a strong homoerotic element even if this was concealed. Edward Albee's *Who's Afraid of Virginia Woolf?* from 1962 seemed to many to be about two homosexual, not heterosexual, couples. The *New York Times* theater critic accused Albee and Williams of "portraying marriage negatively and painting female characters as destroyers and sex maniacs" under the heading "Not What It Seems: Homosexual Motif Gets Heterosexual Guise."

The normalization of homosexual experience is therefore one of the most striking features of the 1950s. This was not only a consequence of Kinsey, though Kinsey helped. Interviews with gay men who went through the fifties indicate that they followed a life course that is recognizable today. One called Louis has described that he "had difficulty deciding which side of the sexual street" he was on. Gay men who came of age at the time struggled to come to terms with their sexuality: "I was depressed when I felt I was gay and pretending to be straight," declared one. They had sex with "straight" guys who were "always talking about girls." They went to homosexual bars for casual sex and to form relationships. Perhaps they learned from an older man. Very often they did not come to terms with themselves until they were well into their thirties. The evidence of the time reveals that homosexual men went through all the same kinds of experiences they have today. Yet there was already a very different attitude from that of Victorian times. Now getting married was not compulsory; finding a permanent male partner without getting married had become a real option. Americans already divided themselves into heterosexual and homosexual, though few could yet admit to the latter identity. And now, unlike in Victorian times, a homosexual person might be either masculine or feminine in appearance.

Perhaps the most striking indicator of the coming of age of homosexual culture in the United States in the fifties was the development of a pornography industry. Robert Mizer's Athletic Model Guild was set up in 1945 (and closed only in 1993). Just as Kinsey obsessively took sexual histories, Mizer took photographs of boys and men. By the 1980s the records of the Guild contained more than six thousand photographs of all sorts of young men whom Mizer had met at gyms, on the beach, and in bus stations, and who had agreed to appear in photographs and stills wearing only the obligatory fig leaf. These young men included cowboys, GIs, athletes, and leather and motorcycle types—they ran the gamut of the American male. Nor was the Guild the only prominent studio devoted to muscular men. Tom of Finland particularly identified a style of gay ideal that was both innocent and erotic. The resulting photos were published in a wide range of magazines from *Physique Pictorial* to *Vim* to *Adonis* to *Tomorrow's Man*. These essentially homoerotic magazines were, however, read widely because of widespread interest in body-building. And they gained mainstream visibility with the help of Mae West who in 1954 decided to replace her chorus of half-naked girls with half-naked musclemen. When in 1955 West and Jayne Mansfield engaged in a public cat fight over one of them—Mr. Universe, Mickey Hargitay—there was further publicity for the genre.

All of this suggested the mainstreaming of gay male experience. But what of lesbians? Essentially the same patterns recurred as in the 1920s: a middle-class respectable world of love and ritual and a rough and tough working-class underworld, which has recently been illuminated by Elizabeth Kennedy and Madeleine Davis in a study of Buffalo, New York. Working-class lesbians embarked on a bizarre imitation of heterosexual relations. Several women would dress as men: "I looked funny trying to look like a man. Man's pants look funny because I'm very short-waisted and big-busted," reminisced Pat Bond in the 1970s film *The Word Is Out* about her life as a "butch." Such women were expected to imitate male behavior. They should be aggressive and make the advances, and they should always treat the "femmes" as ladies. The femmes, on the other hand, should always *be* ladies. They should dress in women's clothing, which meant they should have the celebrated "sweater" style of contemporary film stars, and they should always be passive.

These styles were played out in various obscure bars across the nation. But lesbianism was more widely diffused than ever before. The vogue for lesbian pulp fiction of the fifties and sixties aimed at titillating heterosexual males, but novels such as *Queer Patterns* and *The Sex Between* exposed what was regarded as deviancy to an ever-wider audience. Middle-class lesbians, however, prided themselves on their discretion. Their organizations, such as the Daughters of Bilitis, and its newspaper *The Ladder*, advocated a kind of continuation of the old Victorian female world. They were certainly no rebels as they insisted on "advocating a mode of behavior and dress acceptable to society." In their journals the middle-class women railed at "butches" who seemed to them to look "stereotypically like males." By the same token, young working-class lesbians who followed the butch/femme model referred disparagingly to these middle-class lesbians as "kikis," whom they accused of buckling under by dressing like conventional women.

Hence the 1950s consisted of a wider and more varied sexual culture than had perhaps ever existed in the United States. The need for strong cultural cohesion in order to fight communism influenced the great societal emphasis on the traditional American family in these years. Yet equally the phenomenal strength of the American economy encouraged a carefully packaged sexual rebellion if it made sense commercially—hence the relative freedom given to youth and the popularity of youth films and rock 'n' roll. In the growing atmosphere of toleration, homosexuality flourished as did the sexually subversive Beat writers. In this way the 1950s contained the seeds and birth pangs of the decades to follow.

6

The Sexual Revolution of the 1960s and 1970s

THE 1950s had seen both a revival of traditional neo-Victorian family values and a rebellion against them boosted by a highly consumption-oriented youth culture. In the 1960s the consumer boom continued. As the baby-boom generation, born after World War II, came of age, they formed a higher proportion of the population than ever before. Americans in the sixties faced the great moral challenges posed by the civil rights movement and the Vietnam War. Some sought to build the world over as a fairer and more just place. In this heady atmosphere, the young created their own countercultural movements in the universities. The sixties youth movements believed that the dominant family values of American society—that is, Victorian morality—helped preserve a system they regarded as rotten. Therefore youth must try to change their personal lives. The growth of sexual freedom was vital if Americans were to be liberated from oppressive traditions. Frequent sex was thus an expression of one's personal freedom. Feelings such as jealousy and practices like monogamy were bourgeois; according to this, sex outside of marriage was a revolutionary statement. So, like the Greenwich Village bohemians and the Beats before them, sixties rebels found sex a liberating act. In the process they helped bring to fruition Kinsey's dream of sexual freedom.

The rebels found inspiration in a number of intellectuals who, in the tradition of Havelock Ellis, spread the gospel of sexual liberation. Wilhelm Reich, the post-Freudian psychologist, was a vital influence on many thinkers; the cultural historian Warren Susman went so far as to call the 1960s "the decade of Wilhelm Reich." Reich believed that the cause of neurosis was the patient's inability to enjoy sufficiently intense orgasms. He devised his infamous orgone machine in order to help his patients accomplish orgasmic intensity.

Another native German, Herbert Marcuse, was a major figure to the youth counterculture. His works, such as *Eros and Civilization* (1955), were understood to mean that capitalism was best upset by having lots of sex: "the free gratification of man's instinctual needs." This suited radical youth as it gave them justification for what they were doing anyway. Marcuse seemed to raise desire to the level of a revolutionary act. Yet he appeared to have doubts as he realized what he had helped unleash. By 1972 his concept of "repressive tolerance" seemed to suggest that capitalism allowed sexual freedom in order to detract people from serious political action. But by this time Marcuse's influence, like the counterculture, was on the wane.

Norman O. Brown had no such quibbles. He explicitly rejected heterosexuality and monogamy in favor of bisexuality and of what he called "polymorphous perversity" (by which he meant complete sexual satisfaction). He believed that society caused the ego to repress sexual instincts by means of "civilized sexual morality," and that it was necessary to overthrow that morality in order to free the libido. As critic Vance Packard put it, "He proposes a return to a Dionysian world of sensuality and a return to innocence with an emphasis on uninhibited expression of sex."

A now neglected but important figure for rebels was the New York psychologist Albert Ellis, head of the Institute for Rational Living. Following Reich, he argued that "Sex should be fun, and the more sex fun a person has, the sounder he will be psychologically." In *Sex Without Guilt* (1958), Ellis proposed the psychological benefits of this "fun morality": "sexual release, psychological release, sexual competence, ego enhancement, adventure and experience, improved marital selection, heterosexual democratization, decrease in jealousy; sex is fun." Ellis's institute was housed in a New York building that one critic charged with being a "six-story palace to permissiveness."

These intellectuals were influenced to some degree by "growth" or humanistic psychologists such as Carl Rogers, Erich Fromm, and, most important, Abraham Maslow. In their view, the key to psychological health was not adjustment to society as the classical psychoanalysis of Freud had suggested, but individual "growth" and "fulfillment." Such psychologists regarded the family, with its control over morality, as a straitjacket that retarded the individual's development. Individuals should "get in touch" with their feelings to discuss how they felt about this or that, and to act on how they felt regardless of the consequences for others. Feeling good was all that mattered. Repression of instincts would only multiply neuroses. As Della Reese sang in 1972, "If it feels good, do it."

Youth and its mentors did not create the sexual revolution by themselves. A liberalization of the laws on obscenity made possible many new departures. In 1960 federal courts had determined that D. H. Lawrence's *Lady Chatterly's Lover* could not be categorized as obscene. No one seriously doubted that this work was literature, though deeply flawed. The Supreme Court clouded the issue of what was acceptable and what was not by saying that a work was acceptable provided that "prevailing community standards" were not violated. But this would render a great many books obscene. On the other hand, the Supreme Court determined that a work was acceptable if it had "redeeming social value." This would certify a large number of books that had earlier been regarded as obscene. In effect the court's lack of clarity opened the floodgates. Henry Miller's *Tropic of Cancer* finally became widely available. Then, in 1965, Maurice Girodias, whose Olympia Press had earlier been first to publish such works as Vladimir Nabokov's *Lolita*, Lawrence Durrell's *The Black Book,* and Frank Harris's *Life and Loves,* published *The Olympia Reader.* In the introduction to this work, Girodias presented himself as an embattled cultural outlaw in the struggle for freedom of expression. The legal publication of pornography was to be for him the culmination of the rebellion against Victorian morality: "Writing db's [dirty books] was generally considered a professional exercise as well as a necessary participation in the fight against the Square World—an act of duty." He continued: "The colorful banner of pornography was as good as any other to rally the rebels: the more ludicrous the form of the revolt, the better it was, as a revolt against ordinary logic, and ordinary good taste, restraint, and current morals." Hence Girodias, with unintended help from the Supreme Court, put pornography fairly and squarely in its true context, on the leading edge of the attack on traditional values.

By 1965 such a frank admission was possible. That year, in the case of *A Book named "John Cleland's Memoirs of a Woman of Pleasure" et al. v. Attorney General of Massachusetts,* the Supreme Court gave its stamp of approval to the novel *Fanny Hill.* The court found it of "literary, historical, and social importance," which meant that it could not be said to be "utterly without redeeming social value." The defense had cleverly employed a number of English professors to vouch for the work as literature. One of them suggested that Fanny Hill was an "intellectual," that the work was "well-written." Another claimed that the book should be published purely because it was "widely accredited as the first deliberately dirty novel in English." And even in those cases where obscenity charges were upheld, the justices could not agree on a definition of "obscenity." This just added to the confusion about what was appropriate in public and what not. And into the void the boundaries of acceptability could be extended further. Thus the groundwork was laid for a new respectability for pornography. Within a short while, anything was freely available, "from the Marquis de Sade on down." In 1970 the President's Commission on Pornography recommended still further toleration. According to the historian William O'Neill, an Ivy League bookshop now placed all the hottest work from publishers on a rack bluntly titled "Dirty Books." The way was open for the establishment in the 1970s of the popularly named "dirty bookstore," usually concreted over but with bright lights inside. Invariably, as the volume and variety of pornography increased, these bookstores set themselves up in main shopping thoroughfares next to McDonald's. By the 1980s, leather-jacketed sociology professors could take their students on research trips to such places.

As tolerance of pornography grew, so writers of literature and of plays dared to become much more explicit. This trend had been building throughout the century. Philip Roth scored with *Portnoy's Complaint* (1969), a luridly described account of one man's obsession with masturbation. Similarly explicit was John Updike's *Rabbit, Run* (1960). But it was Norman Mailer who excelled himself in a 1971 polemic, *The Prisoner of Sex,* where he lashed out in filthy language in order to express his anger at the emerging feminist movement. Defending Henry Miller from an assault by the feminist Kate Millett, Mailer insisted on the worth of primeval and unreformed male sexuality. In the theatre, two musicals especially extended the boundaries. The hugely successful 1969 musical *Hair* saw the whole cast removing their clothes. *Hair* was followed in 1970 by the similarly successful and similarly scandalous *Oh! Cal-cutta!* which was performed in the nude.

The early 1960s saw several further challenges to Holly-wood's production code, as the commercially driven studios sought ways to build their profits by extending the boundaries of taste. Many of the early challenges came from abroad—from Europe and especially Britain—before Hollywood began to join in by mid-decade. In 1961, Dirk Bogarde's *The Victim* caused a stir with its positive portrayal of homosexual-ity. According to the rigors of the code, homosexuality was al-ways to be punished. And *The Victim* certainly followed that guideline. Yet Bogarde's character, a lawyer whose career is threatened by the blackmail threats of a young man, is pre-sented quite sympathetically. Bogarde himself summed up the film's significance: "It was the first film in which a man said I love you to another man."

At the turn of the decade, other films from Europe chal-lenged the production code. The great Italian filmmaker Fed-erico Fellini portrayed in *La Dolce Vita* (1960) an intellectual murdering his children. Hollywood columnist Hedda Hopper remarked of the film that "It features homosexuals, lesbians, a wealthy nymphomaniac, aimless artists, and repulsive orgies too sordid to write about." Yet it was Louis Malle's *The Lovers* that got into trouble with the law. In 1959 it was confiscated by Cleveland police. Eventually, in a landmark decision, the Supreme Court overturned a lower court's judgment of ob-scenity.

By this time the production code was crumbling. Stanley Kubrick's film of Vladimir Nabakov's controversial novel of underage sex, *Lolita*, received production code approval in May 1961 only when it was agreed that Lolita would be fifteen years old in the film (she had been twelve in the book). Kubrick himself noted that "it allows pants to come down but never to fall." But it was an extremely risqué film all the same. And, having passed it, the Production Code Administration forfeited a great deal of credibility.

Thus many movies in the early to mid-1960s dared to go further. It is hard to believe today, but the early James Bond films were then judged bold. As played by Sean Connery, Bond upset American ideas of the stereotypical repressed English gentleman by presenting him as a caddish lover and playboy. The series also loved sexually titillating scenes: in *Goldfinger* (1964) a laser beam almost emasculates Bond, and Goldfinger's secretary is stripped and painted gold all over so that she dies of suffocation. The 1964 Oscar-winning movie *Tom Jones* heralded a new wave of British films that indulged in uninhibited realism. This movie of Henry Fielding's eighteenth-century novel is a tale of a rake's adventures without an overt moral message: Jones is presented affectionately. Although there are no explicit sex scenes in the film, there is much eroticism when Tom Jones (played by Albert Finney) and Jenny Jones (Joyce Redman) look into each other's eyes while they rip food apart and stuff it into each other's faces. As the code lost its grip, portrayals of female characters became more daring. Raquel Welch in *One Million Years B.C.* (1966) romped around scantily clad; more subtle was Elizabeth Taylor's famous bathing scene in *Cleopatra* (1963).

In 1965, Sidney Lumet's *The Pawnbroker,* a psychological study of a Nazi concentration camp survivor, brought the crisis over movie censorship to a head. This was obviously a film of deep moral seriousness. Of necessity it required women to expose their breasts in a scene where the pawnbroker comes across a prostitute who reminds him of the abuse his wife had endured from the Nazis. Lumet fought and won a fierce battle with the Production Code Administration to get the picture passed. But the film was so obviously in violation of the code that by passing it the PCA helped bring about its own demise.

Everywhere the forces of censorship were losing out in the mid-1960s. The Legion of Decency, long the scourge of liberals, closed its doors, its chief declaring that "nudity on the screen would soon become as common as blowing your nose." For by this time the calls for liberalization were reaching a crescendo. One magazine editor wrote that he looked forward "to the day when all motion picture producers will stop hiding behind Victorian skirts." Calls such as this led initially to a revised code in which the major innovation was the recommendation of an M rating for some films—"suggested for mature audiences."

In 1966 the director Mike Nichols's *The Graduate* was a mainstream hit that gauged how far the public's tolerance had reached. In this movie Dustin Hoffman, in his film debut, played Benjamin, a rather shy young college graduate who is expected by his family and friends to "get going" with his life and become a respectable businessman. But then he is seduced by one of his parents' best friends, played by Anne Bancroft. Hoffman then falls in love with her daughter Katherine, and after a period of trying to maintain a relationship with both, he chooses the daughter. In one of many hilarious scenes, Bancroft hitches up her skirts, promising sex with Hoffman. But Nichols insisted he had a moral purpose in directing the film: "I think Benjamin and Katherine will end up exactly like their parents. That's what I'm trying to say in the last scene." But the movie was not interpreted that way: the young people's relationship was seen as an act of resistance by two people who would otherwise be totally at the mercy of their parents' manipulation.

Movies could now with ease become more daring. Free rein could be given to a moviemaker's agenda. The director of *The*

Trip (1967), a film aimed at the emerging youth culture, wrote that "It's very important that every fifteen pages or so there be a touch of nudity. It keeps the audience interested." The film was simply packed with nudity. This gained the *Los Angeles Times*'s approval: "There hasn't been such textual richness on a screen since the heyday of Joseph von Sternberg." The 1968 Italian film *Blow Up,* featuring Vanessa Redgrave and David Hemmings, included full frontal nudity for the first time. This film by the Italian director Michelangelo Antonioni was the tale of a young photographer (Hemmings) who snapped his way round swinging London, effortlessly gliding through a world of parties, drugs, and models. Dave Greenberg of *Voice of America* declared the movie to be "moral junk masquerading as realism, little more than a stag film rocked up as art." *Variety* also compared it to a "stag film." The Motion Picture and Broadcasters Association refused to give it their seal of approval. MGM, however, was aggressively determined to have the film released. So the studio found a loophole: they resuscitated a subsidiary through which they were able to release the movie without a production code seal of approval. Other studios now followed MGM's lead, releasing controversial material through subsidiaries.

Mainstream movies too grew ever more bold as the studios sought to enlarge their audiences. Warren Beatty ushered in a new era of daring with *Bonnie and Clyde* (1967), who had been real-life 1930s outlaws but were now repackaged as youth-generation rebels: "We are young. We are in love. We kill people." *I, A Woman* exposed as much of the leading lady as the law allowed, so that the police were unable to press charges when asked to. By 1969, Ken Russell's *Women in Love* was able to be released despite the director's blunt affirmation that he wanted "to shake people up . . . [he] wanted to shake people into life."

The production code was now effectively useless. A new X

rating was introduced in 1969 with the industry's assurance that "We believe in self-restraint and self-regulation in the American tradition." In effect the introduction of the X rating meant that movie censorship, at least for the purpose of maintaining boundaries for adults, was dead. The rating got off to a good start with John Schlesinger's *Midnight Cowboy* (1969), a complex story of a homosexual hustler which one critic described as dignifying the "X classification as a work of artistic integrity." But the rating soon grew into disrepute with the 1970 release of Mike Sarne's film of Gore Vidal's comic spoof of sex-change operations, *Myra Breckinridge*. And the rating lost credibility further when Russ Meyer's pornographic *Vixen!* (1968) earned literally millions (it had cost only $75,000 to make) when given the rating. "X" simply became associated with sexploitation.

Other areas of culture fueled the changes. Radical new fashions for women came across from Britain. Rising hemlines brought the miniskirt, which caused a great stir in 1965 when it first appeared. Only when Jacqueline Onassis was spotted wearing one did they become more respectable. From 1966 to 1968 the microskirt entered into vogue while the British model Twiggy, skinny as a rake and sixteen, the exact opposite of previous ideals of femininity, became a star. Controversy also surrounded the ever skimpier bikini swimsuit. The critic Vance Packard observed that it "greatly broadens the area of the female body where it is permissible to engage in casual petting, even in public." But it was men's clothing that most upset Packard. He noted what he called "the dandified look" which came in with the Beatles. He observed, in horror, that "Many young Englishmen began wearing eyebrow makeup, transparent lipstick, billowy satin shirts with floral patterns, fluffed-up hair, high-heeled boots, and lots of jewelry. One male musical group, the Pretty Things, had pink-dyed hair." The writer Tom Wolfe remarked that "Suddenly

mankind were bursting out of the traditional old gray business sack suits like a bunch of randy roosters." These styles
sifted across from the trendy world of "Swinging London"
where fashion designers, gay and straight, mixed with rock
stars, actors, and other media folk and sought to spread a
gospel of greater sexual freedom.

Since the 1920s advertisers had used sex to sell. But now
they could be much more blatant in their imagery. Advertising also surged beyond previous boundaries. Packard, still
horrified, noted that by 1966 sales of male cosmetics had
reached $500 million. Their aim was to enhance sexual attrac-
tiveness. The president of the Mennen Company said that the
key question to ask of cosmetics was, "Will the girls like it?"
Therefore advertisers determined to show in their advertising
that the girls would. Aztec, a fragrance for men, produced
three provocative pictures of a couple which they dubbed "Before," "During," and "After." Piping Rock aftershave featured
an ad with a girl cooing, "Was it him—or his Piping Rock?"
Product development departments meanwhile strove to find a
spray that would break down women's inhibitions once and
for all. The trend was clear: clothing and styles for both men
and women became more and more sexualized as fashion influenced and was influenced by the burgeoning youth culture.

Rock music was, however, to have the most influence on
the mood of the young. The standard account is that after the
army Elvis had lost his edge and that American rock was
cleaned up and sanitized as stars such as Bobby Vee and
Frankie Avalon watered down its impact. Elvis may have returned from the army with the uninspiring and derivative single "Stuck on You," but his comeback album *Elvis Is Back*
(1960) really rocked out. Elvis never lost his popularity in
these years, and if he had lost the power to shock, he was still
capable of rocking. Nor was he alone. Early sixties American

pop had a rock 'n' roll teenage vitality that could rival the 1950s. Record company talent scouts sought out good-looking young men to spread the gospel of liberation via rock. One of the most popular groups was Dion and the Belmonts, white Doo Wop imitators from the Bronx. They scored their two biggest hits at the end of 1961 with two songs that defined teenage rebellion from parental morality. "Runaround Sue" is a very male look at a bad girl and lyrically expresses peer-group attitudes to sex: "Keep away from Runaround Sue." But it was okay for a man to run around: the Belmonts' next song "The Wanderer," captures this double standard in action. Dion is the "type of guy who likes to roam around." He "can never settle down." As soon as a girl suggests that he does he "[hops] right into that car of mine and [drives] around the world." One could find such frank lyrics all over the rhythm-and-blues and country charts, but no mainstream popular song had so swaggeringly defined male sexual rebellion in this way.

The same realism was present in the Brill Building writers of the early to mid-1960s who brought a new lyrical sophistication to rock. Gerry Goffin and Carole King especially evoked a teenage anxiety that reflected their own experience of a volatile and passionate love affair. Their song for the Shirelles, "Will You Love Me Tomorrow?" laid the issue of premarital sex straight on the line: "Tonight you're mine completely/But will you love me tomorrow?" As the rock historian Ed Ward explained it, "Clearly the girl was going to give in, endangering her reputation, but she was willing to take the risk because she loved her boyfriend." Other Goffin and King songs were easily dismissed as shallow and sugary because of the orchestration and vocal delivery. Yet they could be equally as honest. "Up on the Roof," a hit for the Drifters, describes where many teenagers had to go for privacy, while "Go Away

Little Girl," a hit for Steve Lawrence, took up a real dilemma in the open teen culture of the time where sex was legal only at the age of sixteen.

The early 1960s also saw one of the greatest of all dance crazes, the Twist. Supposedly invented by black homosexuals, this dance involved no physical touching, but its hip-shaking intensity imitated the sex act. When Dick Clark first saw it being performed on his show, he shouted, "For God's sake keep the cameras off that couple!" But the dance soon spread. An easy dance to perform, it became popular with older couples, and its popularity lasted until the British invasion of 1964. Yet it stayed controversial. The choreographer Geoffrey Holder described it as "sex turned into a disgusting spectator sport." The writer Beverly Nichols commented that "the essence of the Twist, the curious perverted heart of it, is that you dance it alone." The British rock critic George Melly noted that "Danced by the young it is certainly immensely erotic, but danced, and danced badly, by the middle-aged it becomes obscene." No wonder that President Eisenhower observed with characteristic wryness of the fad, "I have no objection to the Twist, but it does represent some kind of change in our standards. What has happened to our concepts of beauty and morality?"

The British invasion of the mid-sixties changed rock music forever. These pop groups, like the films and fashions that were coming out of Swinging London, showed little reverence for traditional values. They were often managed, and even manufactured, by homosexual svengali like Brian Epstein, who felt little loyalty to family values and even less if there was money to be made from sexually subversive songs and behavior. When the Beatles landed in New York in February 1964 they revived the hysteria that had greeted previous teen idols such as Elvis Presley and Pat Boone. Yet they were cleverly presented as thoroughly clean-cut young men. Their popularity therefore soon went beyond their initial teen fans and expanded to include a much broader audience. The Beatles' songs, even as they ranged beyond the previous boundaries of rock music, both lyrically and musically usually remained wholesome—except when drugs intervened.

The songs of the Rolling Stones—who soon approached the Beatles in popularity—were another matter. Nor were they mere stooges of record company bosses. Intelligent, middle class, and well educated, they knew how far they could go. Hence they carefully planned the image of rebellion that the title of the band suggested. They did not, for example, release their raunchiest number, "Little Red Rooster," as a single in the United States, instead preferring the prophetic "Time Is on My Side." And their first American No. 1, "Satisfaction," is a brilliant lyric about a young man confused and frustrated by the sexual demands of modern society. But with time they became more daring. Their ponderously titled, poorly produced, yet underestimated pop-Freudian "Have You Seen Your Mother, Baby, Standing in the Shadows?" went so far as to feature the band members in drag on the record cover. It was the 1970s before the Stones could be as bold as they wished, but in the 1960s they helped set the mood of intelligent liberation. It was a measure of changing mores.

Other members of the British invasion similarly dabbled with what was then called deviancy. The married and heterosexual Kinks enjoyed pretending they were ambiguous in their sexual preferences. Nevertheless they helped to pioneer gay rock in their 1965 minor hit "See My Friend," in which the singer declares his intention to "see my friend" "way across the river." And they posed for one publicity photograph with horsewhips.

By the late sixties there were even more sexually subversive undercurrents in rock. The Doors were perhaps the most controversial of all rock groups. They were led by Jim Morrison, an exhibitionist poseur who claimed he could maintain an erection for the course of a two-hour performance. He had no doubts about where it was at: "We make concerts sexual politics. The sex starts with me, and then moves out to include the charmed circle of musicians on stage. The music we make goes out to the audience and interacts with them: they go home and interact with the rest of reality, so the whole sex thing turns out to be one big ball of fire." After Morrison, the sexual aspects of rock, so intrinsic to the form anyway, could no longer be concealed, any more than Morrison was able to hide his member during performances.

Behavior and attitudes still lagged behind popular culture, but important changes were afoot. The availability of the contraceptive pill beginning in 1961 was the linchpin of the sexual revolution because it made the divorce of sex from procreation so easy. Planned Parenthood clinics now mushroomed throughout the United States, encouraged by a federal government worried about population growth, especially among the poor. Here doctors, in stark contrast to their Victorian forebears, largely ignored any moral issues that the Pill raised. Doctor Dale Clinton of Lawrence, Kansas, for example, declared, "Our job is simply to give them what they ask for . . . and we do not attempt to educate the women." As one study of Lawrence has shown: "With virtually no exceptions, women seeking contraceptives at the health department came away with the pill."

The journalist Helen Gurley Brown soon realized the Pill's significance. In 1963 she published *Sex and the Single Girl*. More than any other book, it heralded the most significant aspect of the renewed sexual revolution—the growing freedom of women. Brown celebrated the joys of "the single, urban, working girl," whom she described as "the newest glamour girl of our times." She compared the single girl favorably to a married woman: "she is not a parasite, a dependent, a scrounger, a sponger, a dependent, or a bum" who needed a man around the whole time. Brown, who soon converted her insights into the editorship of *Cosmopolitan* magazine and made it a multi-million-dollar success, understood very well that the keystone of women's emerging sexual freedom was that they should be as free to behave badly as men had always been: "Nice girls DO have affairs and they do not necessarily die of them."

A growing understanding of women's physiology aided their "liberation." The psychologist Judd Marmor in 1954 had "discovered" the clitoral orgasm. But word of its existence spread when sexologists William Masters and Virginia Johnson in 1966 published *Human Sexual Response*. They described in great detail what they had learned through numerous observations of the sex act. If science had had any doubt in Victorian times that women were orgasmic, now all doubt was readily allayed. Not only was women's capacity for orgasm based in the clitoris, but women were discovered to have many different orgasmic responses and were even able to have multiple orgasms! Masters and Johnson's book reads at times almost like a parody of Kinsey, whose work they took to its logical conclusion by arguing that, effectively, sex was purely for pleasure.

Ideas like this soon dominated advice literature. The explicit manual *The Sensuous Woman* (1969) was filled with advice about the clitoral orgasm. If the clitoris was the site of women's orgasmic power, other types of sex, apart from the missionary position, might be recommended. J, the pseudonym of the author, therefore explicitly praised oral sex. Of anal sex she was more cautious: "Cheer up, this is optional." J usually recommended sex between any two people, though she also casually advised orgies, as if they differed little from

Tupperware parties ("If you go, don't wear a good dress"). J also recommended wife-swapping and "swinging." Her book not only divorced sex from procreation but from all emotion.

J's book went on to sell nine million copies and set the tone for the best-selling sex manual of the seventies, *The Joy of Sex* by British sexologist Alex Comfort. Published in 1972, it continued the trend by stressing the equality of different types of sex. Sex was no different from choosing from an array of menus. All that really mattered was what produced the greatest pleasure: in the same book, advice for virgins could be found alongside information about heterosexual sado-masochism and pictures of men and women having sex. These manuals by Comfort and J were the inspiration for Shere Hite's 1976 *Hite Report* on women's sexuality, an impassioned plea for women to insist that men give them orgasms. Presented in the guise of sex research, Hite had actually placed ads in pornographic magazines requesting that people fill out her questionnaire. Needless to say, the women who responded advocated sexual liberation. The *Report* is therefore now regarded by sociologists as a classic example of a skewed sample. Yet it reflected the new assertiveness of women and their demands for sexual pleasure.

The popularity of these books suggests that Americans in general were increasingly open to the new morality. Entrepreneurial elites had financed and created a popular culture that broke taboos and expanded boundaries in order to sell its products. Intellectuals, psychologists, and experts in sexuality justified this freewheeling morality in their writings that, as affluence grew, found an ever more willing youth prepared to break with the past. But did the sexual revolution have much meaning beyond the self-consciously radical youth culture? In the 1960s older values still held sway. There was a lag between the expanding boundaries of popular culture and the values and behavior adhered to by many Americans. Even as late as

1970 one survey suggested that half of Americans believed that premarital sex was always unacceptable. Any new sexual morality in the late sixties was, according to the pollster Daniel Yankelovich, "confined to a minority of college students." But other studies suggest that permissive attitudes were growing among younger groups.

Changes in behavior were hard to pinpoint. One study indicated that the number of men having premarital intercourse did not increase between 1965 and 1970, though the number of women so involved did. Attitudes changed more than behavior. In those five years, those who regarded sex before marriage as "immoral" actually dropped by half. Further, disapproval of multiple sex partners fell by a third. Between 1971 and 1975 behavior changes seem to have caught up a little. There was a dramatic rise of 14 percent in the number of men who had sex before marriage, and an astonishing increase of 54 percent for women. This surely reflected changing attitudes. In 1959 a Roper Poll had shown that only 22 percent of respondents approved of premarital intercourse. By 1975, in a similar poll, approval was as high as 58 percent.

And Americans were having sex when younger. One study of high school males between 1970 and 1973 indicates that the number having sexual intercourse went up from 27.8 percent to 33.4 percent, and for girls from 16.1 percent to 22.4 percent. By the mid-seventies about one-third of high school senior girls had already had sexual intercourse. Dating was being replaced by mixed-sex interaction among peers, a system so casual it discouraged taboos but encouraged "going all the way." A 1976 survey by Melvin Zelnik and John F. Kantner of the sexual behavior of adolescent girls indicated that having lots of dates was linked to high levels of premarital intercourse. The dating system had in fact begun to lose many of its functions. Peers now accepted fewer limitations on sexual behavior, which removed much of the purpose of dating. In the

permissive society, personal growth was not supposed to be
hindered by sexual repression of any kind. And by the 1970s
the ideas of the "me" generation stressed that it was no one
else's business what you did in bed—not your parents, and
certainly not your peers. Young Americans' sexual attitudes
now truly resembled sociologist Ira Reiss's idea of "permissiveness with affection." Affection justified intercourse. John
DeLamater and Patricia MacCorquodale's 1973 study of Wis-
consin youth confirmed their thinking: only one in ten believed in chastity before marriage. Yet perhaps the strongest
sign of change in American moral standards were the one-
third in this study who believed that "sex without affection
with mutual consent" was acceptable.

Illustrative of this trend was the growth of a "singles culture." In 1964 the first singles bar opened on New York's
Upper East Side. Soon such bars appeared throughout the
country. With the advent of the Pill, the successful treatment
of venereal diseases, and the liberalization of abortion laws,
apartment complexes and singles clubs proliferated. The sociologist Robert Staples examined the African-American singles
scene in the mid-seventies and revealed the aimlessness and
frustration of this world. One young man noted that he'd
"never met a woman I'd like to spend the rest of my life with.
I've never discovered commitment or how to make it to a
woman." A female engineer declared that she "love[d] being
single, since I was tied down to school so long. It feels good
now to be free and to be promiscuous, in addition to feeling I
have no commitments to anyone but myself." As Staples himself noted of the scene, "It seems that love and romantic relationships have become just one more commodity in a material
society. If you do not like it, return it in two years."

But how promiscuous were Americans really? The image
of the 1960s/1970s youth culture implies that they were very
promiscuous indeed. But in fact they weren't. A study con-

ducted in the early 1990s suggests that among those in their fifties, who had missed the "sexual revolution," about 37 percent had had just one partner in their lives. Among those who had come of age in the sixties, about 24 percent had had just one partner in their lives. Those with two to four partners remained about the same percentage regardless of age. Those with ten to twenty partners rose from 8 percent to 12 percent, while those with multiple partners increased from 8 percent to about 13 percent. Here was tangible, real change, but it was scarcely revolutionary. It suggests that for all the changes in attitudes and popular culture, behavioral change was limited.

Marriage, though, became a less attractive option. Americans married at an increasingly later age. The perception grew that "one lost freedom in marriage." This explains the growth in popularity in the 1970s of "cohabitation" or "living together." A 1974 college survey noted that 29 percent of men and 18 percent of women had already lived with someone of the other sex. This was confirmed by a mid-seventies survey that showed 33 percent of men and 25 percent of women as having lived at some time with someone they were involved with sexually. For many couples, cohabitation replaced the age-old tradition of engagement. A study concluded that "By 1975, at a given moment, one in seven young people 20 to 24 years old were living together." A recent study has shown that the percentage of first partnerships that were marriages was 84.5 percent for men and 93.8 percent for women among those born between 1933 and 1942, but was down to 46.6 percent of men and 57.3 percent of women among those born between 1943 and 1952. And this trend was accelerated because as colleges expanded, more and more students lived off campus with boyfriends or girlfriends. This phenomenon, previously largely regarded as working class, gained ground across the whole social structure. Yet while "living together" superficially resembled a marital relationship, according to one study "Cohabitation led to marriage in a bit over one in three cases" only. Thus in the 1970s sexual revolution, as young people claimed greater autonomy over their life choices than ever before, they chose to expand the established phase of "going steady" by moving in together away from parents. This was an important change, because it suggested, as Staples had noted of African Americans, that young people could simply choose to drop each other—just as they could with any other commodity—as they grew bored.

The growth in the divorce rate crowned the permissive society. The development of "no-fault" divorce probably contributed. This tactic began with the Family Law Act of 1969 in California, approved by its governor, the divorced (and re-married) Ronald Reagan. In place of the previous seven grounds for divorce, there were now only two: the vaguely titled "irremediable breakdown of marriage" and "incurable insanity." Other states followed California's lead so that by mid-1977 only three states lacked "no-fault" divorce laws. Yet "no-fault" divorce was insufficiently radical for many who argued that it only put in place what judges had been practicing for some time. Several hippies preferred "contract marriages." For example, to cite one case, they might agree to marry for ten years and then decide if they wished to part. Others argued for a system of "divorce on demand" by which divorce would automatically be granted. No wonder that in the 1970s the United States became renowned for its divorce rate. In the decade one in three American marriages ended in divorce. One British wit described the United States as "the land where everybody is divorced once at twelve and five times by the age of twenty-one."

If the white family was in a bad way, the plight of African Americans was worse. In the fall of 1965 Daniel Patrick Moynihan published *The Negro Family: The Case for Affirma-*

tive Action. The report was a sensation in its devastating claim that "The evidence—not final, but powerfully persuasive—is that the Negro family in the urban ghettoes is crumbling." While the black middle-class family remained relatively stable, for poor African Americans "the fabric of conventional social relationships has all but disintegrated." The figures were indeed stunning. Illegitimacy among blacks had risen from 16.8 percent in 1940 to 23.6 percent in 1963, compared to a rise from only 2 percent to 3 percent among whites. Twenty-one percent of black women headed families compared to 9 percent among white women, and the figure was rising. Twenty-five percent of black women were divorced, separated, or living away from their husbands. Among African Americans, it seemed, the decline of the family was more advanced.

There was still one more twist: the feminist reaction to the sexual revolution, which now gathered speed. The response to Betty Friedan's *The Feminine Mystique* was so enormous that in 1966 she and a number of other women formed the National Organization for Women (NOW) to lobby for the improvement of women's position in American society. Those who were also involved in the civil rights movement worked hard to undermine divisions of race but in the process uncovered divisions of their own: the male activists in the movement shared traditional attitudes toward women. Stokely Carmichael famously remarked that "The only position for women in our movement is prone." The historian Staughton Lynd has suggested the full extent of the sexism: "Every black SNCC worker with perhaps a few exceptions counted it as a notch on his gun to have slept with a white woman—as many as possible. And I think that was very traumatic for the women who encountered that who hadn't thought that was what going South was about. . . ." On the other hand, as activists Barbara Ehrenreich and Deirdre English had a much more positive experience: "My recollection of it was that it was not an unmitigated disaster. The sexism was there but women were actually having more sexual experience of different kinds and enjoying it. Women were experiencing more sex that was not for procreation and claiming the right to it as well as paying a lower social and emotional cost."

But women had had sufficient bad experiences to begin to join together in making sense of what had happened to them. They were upset with their subordinate position: why should they have to make coffee and not policy? Surely if women were fighting to end one form of oppression they should not be made victims of another. They excluded men from conferences: "the women have asked all the men to leave the stage except for the Vietnam vet who has earned the right to be there." And their vehemence was most strongly reserved for the political left. Shulamith Firestone wrote a letter to the *Guardian:* "You will come around when you have to because you need us more than we need you. . . . The message being Fuck off Left. You can examine your navel from now on. We're starting our own movement." Using insights they had gained from the civil rights movement, many former civil rights activists met together in various "consciousness-raising" groups where they tried to compare experiences with men. Too often this confirmed their prejudices. Influenced by the civil rights movement, they coined the phrase "the personal is political," by which they meant that their relationships with men and with one another reflected and affected how power was organized in society. By changing the relations between men and women, they thought, the whole pattern of male dominance and female subordination in society could be altered. This was important: by politicizing personal life, feminists removed one of Victorianism's key tenets, the need for privacy to preserve sex as extraordinary.

But the radical feminist wave bore on. To illustrate their

position, in 1968 a group of feminists led by Robin Morgan "zapped" the Miss America pageant, crowning a live sheep and hurling what they argued were "objects of female torture," such as copies of the *Ladies' Home Journal*, girdles, and, most famously, bras to show the sexual objectification of women's bodies: "Gentlemen, I offer you the 1969 model. She's better every year. She walks. She talks. She smiles on cue. And she does housework."

Feminism was deeply ambiguous about the sexual revolution. On the one hand, it liberated women to explore their sexuality. On the other hand, heterosexual sex involved consorting with the enemy, with men. Permissiveness generally won out. Kate Millett's *Sexual Politics* (1970) called for a "permissive single standard of sexual freedom." Shulamith Firestone, in her classic polemic *The Dialectic of Sex* (1969), celebrated sex as "life-affirming." The 1973 feminist guide to women's bodies, *Our Bodies, Ourselves,* declared that "[Sex] is a vital physical expression of attachments to other human beings. It is communication that is fun and playful, serious and passionate."

Germaine Greer's *The Female Eunuch* (1970) denounced the historical denial of female sexuality. Being a woman meant being "without libido" and therefore "incomplete, subhuman, a cultural reduction of human possibilities." Greer's work was a witty, and scholarly, call to recognize women as sexual beings, entirely in tune with the mood of the sexual revolution. But she criticized the major new finding on women's sexuality, the clitoral orgasm. For her, the clitoral orgasm made women's sexuality too like men's: "If we localize female response in the clitoris we impose on women the same limitation of sex which has stunted the male response." This meant that sex became mere "masturbation in the vagina." Greer argued that "women's continued high enjoyment of sex, which continues after orgasm, observed by men with wonder, is not based on the clitoris, which does not respond particularly well to continued stimulus, but in a general sensual response." Greer was not here defending the vaginal orgasm. Rather, she saw women's sexuality as more emotionally complex than American feminists would have it.

Feminist literature especially "liberated" women's sexuality, but with a good deal less humor than Greer. In the early 1970s a whole genre of feminist writings grew that, according to the critic Jane Larkin Crain, featured women who rejected marriage as "calamitous in and of itself, and also symptomatic of the allegedly life-negating absurdities of the entire American condition." Crain noted such works as Alix Shulman's *Memoirs of an Ex-Prom Queen* (1972), Anne Roiphe's *Up the Sandbox!* (1970), Lois Gould's *Such Good Friends* (1970), and, perhaps most shocking, Erica Jong's *Fear of Flying* (1973). Isadora Wing, the heroine of Jong's book, has an affair with an analyst who tries to awaken her from her dull, routine marriage: "I thought of all the cautious good-girl rules I had lived by—the good student, the dutiful daughter, the guilty faithful wife who committed adultery only in her head—and I decided that for once I was going to be brave and follow my feelings no matter what the consequences." This causes her to embark on a "bacchanalian junket" through Europe after she leaves her husband. But the heroine soon realizes that her problem is her dependence on men—"I knew for sure I wasn't going to grovel. But that was all I knew ... it was enough."

If one aspect of the feminist revolt called for giving women the same sexual freedoms that men had always enjoyed, another side was anti-men. Jane Crain discusses how men were stereotyped in the novels: "By and large, they are thoroughgoing cads—surly brutes who take no interest in their children and refuse to participate in the running of their households; who commit adultery and sexually neglect their own wives." Many feminists argued that such stereotyping of men was just revenge for how women had historically appeared in literature.

Many feminist revolutionaries engaged in openly antisocial behavior. Valerie Solanis wrote the SCUM manifesto, a proposed Society for Cutting Up Men, before she shot the artist Andy Warhol. Clearly disturbed, she was the most extreme of feminist authors: in her manifesto she described men as a "biological accident," an "incomplete female . . . an emotional cripple" who suffers from "pussy envy." Solanis's case was nonetheless taken on as a major NOW cause by T. Grace Atkinson, president of the New York chapter and protégé of Betty Friedan (who opposed the move).

Shulamith Firestone's *The Dialectic of Sex* was perhaps the most considered of many anti-male feminist polemics. Firestone identified and critiqued male behaviors that she rightly saw as oppressive to women. She insisted that "Men can't love." From this assumption she developed the concept of patriarchy, which was an attempt to explain how men oppressed women. Firestone, however, weakened her case by playing to her audience. She quoted from various men interviewed by *Screw* magazine: "It is not true that only the external appearance of a woman matters. The underwear is also important." "The girl asked me whether I cared for her mind. I was tempted to say that I cared more for her behind." These quotes are arresting, but the sample is too obviously skewed and anecdotal to be taken seriously.

Concurrently, Kate Millett in *Sexual Politics* devised the concept of "sexism," the means by which the men in Firestone's patriarchy dominated women. She equated the system of male dominance over women with racism, the system of white dominance over black people. The concept of "sexism" stuck. Influenced by Atkinson, Millett called for the abandonment of sex roles and the liberation of all women. Her work was lapped up by women across the English-speaking world.

One consequence of this anti-male rhetoric of the women's movement was a turn toward lesbianism. Kate Millett in 1970 accidentally "came out" as a lesbian, and this caused an initial furor that eventually led to Betty Friedan's resignation from NOW after complaining about the "lavender menace" that threatened to engulf it. Judith Brown explicitly endorsed lesbianism as the logical direction for women involved in the women's movement. Brown believed that married women should take breaks from their marriages to spend time with other women, thus ensuring they were committed to their sex. Ann Koedt's 1971 article on the "Myth of the Vaginal Orgasm" extended the lesbian case. If, as Masters and Johnson had popularized, it was unnecessary for a penis to be present for women to have an orgasm, there was no end to women's sexual possibilities. Koedt and Atkinson held a sex workshop at which women talked of "wonderful, detailed stories about sex," of their sadomasochistic and lesbian fantasies. The article was a revelation for many women. One woman even had to "apologize to [her] sisters" for claiming to have had a vaginal orgasm. The biggest implication of the piece was the boost it gave to a new idea: political lesbianism. Dana Dunsmore suggested that women become celibate instead of "squander[ing] their energy on men and sex." The Radicallesbians group argued that "It is the primacy of women's relations to women that is at the heart of women's liberation and the basis of cultural revolution." It may be that some women were not capable of being sexual lesbians, so they became political lesbians who made their primary commitment to women. As one noted, adamantly: "I'm a lesbian. I don't sleep with women. But I'm a lesbian." In some cases they also became lesbian separatists, seeking to avoid contact with men altogether, to "avoid hassling with men." This proved a boon to those women who did have lesbian tendencies. They could have the best of both worlds: they could have sex and be politically correct feminists all at the same time. This did not mean that all lesbians were feminists or that all feminists were lesbians. But there was certainly a great deal of overlap, especially if the growing band of political lesbians were included.

By the mid-1970s the women's movement could boast a couple of great successes. In 1972 Congress approved the Equal Rights Amendment; and in 1973 the Supreme Court's decision in *Roe v. Wade* effectively made abortion legal. As political gains became harder to win, however, the women's movement turned in on itself. Radical feminism became cultural feminism in the mid-seventies, when much of the early seventies anti-male rhetoric culminated in the development of feminist rape theory. By mid-decade there was much concern about an apparent increase in rape in American society. A few high-profile rapes occurred, notably the horrific 1974 rape of the singer Connie Francis. Susan Brownmiller, in *Against Our Will* (1975), concluded that because men dominated women in society, they saw rape as a natural right. Brownmiller pointed out the hopeless inadequacy of laws against rape. Most states allowed women to be questioned about their sexual pasts. In one state, North Carolina, the only illegal rape was against a virgin. And Brownmiller suggested that rape was actually far more common than was usually thought. But her greatest insight was that rape was not so much an act of sex as an act of violence, of "sexual coercion," the direct result of male dominance over women. Hence, most alarmingly, "normal" men could rape; rape was the main means of male dominance both before and since Victorian patriarchy. What she failed to see was that the increased incidence of rape was a consequence of the breakdown in Victorian morality, not a result of it. The psychologist Lynne Segal has seen this point clearly: "Rather than being the indispensable weapon used by men to ensure the subordination of women, might not rape be the deformed behavior of men accompanying the destabilization of gender relations, and the consequent contradictions and insecurities of male gender identities, now at their peak in modern America?"

By the mid-1970s feminism and the sexual revolution seemed unassailable. But the forces of traditional morality in American society now rallied to become by the late seventies a powerful backlash.

This counterattack had one source in the Roman Catholic church's response to the Pill. At first many in the American church supported the Pill. Its Catholic inventor, Dr. John Rock, felt it was far superior to the rhythm method, which he dubbed "Vatican Roulette." He argued that if the church permitted the rhythm method, it should allow the Pill. A Catholic president, John F. Kennedy, indicated his approval. In his *The Experience of Marriage* (1964), the theologian Michael Novak explained the problems that not using contraceptives could cause. In *Commonweal* magazine in 1964, in a symposium on parenthood, the participants pointed out that the blanket ban on contraception needed to be revised. The most influential work was John Noonan's *Contraception: A History of Its Treatment by the Catholic Theologians and Canonists* (1965), which showed there was nothing sacrosanct in natural law about the church's teaching. It had developed almost accidentally. Others in the church had their doubts. The goal of sex, the church argued, was procreation, and clearly the Pill challenged this view. In order to become Catholic Family of the Year, a coveted award given out by the Christian Family Movement, it helped to have more than twelve children. Yet the church, run by celibates, also regarded celibacy in marriage favorably. The Jesuit John Thomas declared that "it is frequently forgotten that the virtue of chastity . . . applies to married couples as well as to others."

It seemed for a while that Rome would relent and come round in support of the Pill. The momentous Second Vatican Council of the early 1960s, convened by John XXIII and completed by Paul VI, opened up all areas of the church's teaching for debate, including the idea of marriage as a sacrament of love as well as for procreation. Just as the Council drew to a close, Pope Paul VI inaugurated the Pontifical Commission on the Family, Population, and Natality. "A reported eighty percent" of the commission came down in favor of contraception. It seemed as if the battle had been won. Then, dramatically, in 1968 the pope issued the encyclical *Humanae Vitae* which explicitly forbade Roman Catholic couples from using contraceptives and permitted the rhythm method only "for grave reasons." The pope explained that "the moment has not come, for man to entrust to his reason and his will, rather than to the biological rhythms of his organism, the task of regulating birth." The growth of birth control would result in men losing "respect for the woman and . . . come to the point of considering her as a mere instrument of selfish enjoyment."

The encyclical led to a fierce storm of controversy in the American church. American bishops immediately approved it. It was widely seen as a powerful reassertion of orthodoxy and traditional morality in the midst of severe pressures for change. But forty priests protested to Cardinal Patrick O'Boyle of Washington, D.C. Seventy-eighty theology teachers declared it "incompatible with the church's authentic self-awareness as expressed at Vatican II." John Noonan tried ingeniously, but unconvincingly, to reinterpret the meaning of the encyclical. He welcomed it on the grounds that, as intercourse during the safe time of the menstrual cycle was not sinful, Catholics who used contraception then would not subvert the teaching of the pope. But Noonan was heavily criticized for his interpretation. Notre Dame's Charles Rice suggested that "Instead of whining about the Church's stand on contraception and trying to weasel out of it, he ought to say 'Serviam!'—'I will serve'—and devote his considerable talents to advancing the teaching of the Vicar of Christ." The Roman Catholic church, the international defender of traditional morality, had been aroused. Although American Catholics now proceeded to disobey the church's teaching on this issue en masse, the backlash against permissiveness had begun.

As the feminist wave hit high tide with the passage of the Equal Rights Amendment and the *Roe v. Wade* decision, forces of opposition gathered steam. As early as 1968 Richard Nixon had played to "the silent majority" of "Middle America" that yearned for solid traditional standards. But the passage of the ERA galvanized the right, because the amendment, briefly and cogently, was an easy issue around which to rally the right's hostility to feminist gains. At the end of 1972 Phyllis Schlafly, a Catholic, founded the National Committee to Stop the ERA, which aimed to prevent the necessary number of states from ratifying the amendment. Feminists had not reckoned on the emergence of Schlafly, who was a formidable operator, adopting the very same tactics as the feminists: coordination at the grass roots and consciousness-raising.

Schlafly also developed some powerful arguments. The ERA, she maintained, was a threat to the family: "See for yourself the unkempt, the lesbians, the radicals, the socialists." They had rejected the family roles of wife and mother. Schlafly launched a broad attack on feminism's gains. Gloria Steinem's *Ms.* magazine she declared to be "anti-family, anti-children, and pro-abortion. . . . Women's lib is a total assault on the role of the American woman as wife and mother." Others on the right suggested that the result of the ERA would be the legalization of rape and growing acceptance of homosexuality. Pastor Jerry Falwell sent out a questionnaire that caught the mood of the anti-ERA forces. "Do you approve of the ratification of the ERA, which could well lead to homosexual

marriages, unisexual bathrooms, and, of course, the manda-
tory drafting of women for military combat?"

The *Roe v. Wade* decision in 1973 sent shock waves through
Christian churches. James P. McFadden heard the news as his
"Road to Damascus conversion." In 1975 he founded *Human
Life Review* as a central focus for efforts to make abortion illegal on the grounds that it was child killing. Anti-abortion ac-
tivism involved fundamentalist Protestant churches as well as
Catholic. It was seen by many as part and parcel of the same
vogue for selfish individualism and anti-family rhetoric as
equal rights for women. Phyllis Schlafly condemned the ERA
on the grounds that it would further confirm the right to
abortion. In 1976 the anti-abortion movement secured its first
success. Republican Representative Henry Hyde of Illinois
helped pass an amendment that barred Medicaid funds from
being used for abortions for poor women. Then in 1978 Congress stopped federal funding of abortions for all government
employees. The backlash was gaining ground.

Supporters of traditional morality were most appalled,
however, by the emergence of a highly politicized homosexual
community. On June 27, 1969, New York City police raided
the Greenwich Village gay bar, the Stonewall Inn. The
Stonewall was a Mafia-run, low-down dive frequented by
homosexuals. It should have been an easy target. But this time
the patrons fought back. No sooner did the paddy wagons ar-
rive and begin to collect the prisoners than the tense atmosphere exploded into a riot. Homosexuals who for centuries
had meekly submitted to police abuse now fought back in a
barrage of epithets: "Pigs," "Faggot cops," "Gay power." A
Puerto Rican, according to the historian Martin Duberman,
yelled at a policeman: "What you got against faggots? We
don't do you nuthin'." By now the vitriol had turned into a
full-blown riot. As cans and coins, even bricks, were thrown
at the police, they were forced to retreat inside the bar. So ter-

rified were some of the police that one declared, "I had been in combat situations, but there was never any time that I felt more scared than then." The situation grew so out of hand that a tactical patrol force, specially trained riot police, had to be called in. Yet even they could not disperse the crowd, as a group of queens sang:

> We are the Stonewall girls
> We wear our hair in curls
> We wear no underwear
> We show our pubic hair.

Finally, the police swept the streets clear of rioters but not before several injuries had been sustained among rioters and policemen. When the riots continued over the course of the weekend, the scene drew various prominent onlookers to the Village. The poet Allen Ginsberg emerged from the bar and declared the patrons to be "beautiful—they've lost that wounded look faggots had ten years ago." One newspaper referred to the "hairpin drop heard around the world." And the leader of the police operation, Deputy Inspector Seymour Pine, saw the riots as a turning point too: "For those of us in public morals, things were completely changed . . . suddenly they were not submissive anymore."

The Stonewall riots have come to be symbolic of the start of the gay liberation movement that succeeded the homosexual rights movement. And not without reason. But they also represented the culmination of tensions among homosexual Americans that were leading to a growing militancy, rejecting the moderation and respectability of the older homophile movement.

Franklin Kameny had long challenged the bland reformist ethos of the Mattachine Society, the first major homosexual rights organization. Kameny, a trained astronomer who had lost his job in 1957 when it had been discovered that he had a conviction for "lewd conduct," was in no mood for compromise. He rejected the idea that "gay is sick": "the entire movement is going to stand or fall upon the question of whether homosexuality is a sickness and upon our taking a firm stand on it," he said. Kameny had a very positive view of his own homosexuality; later it was he who came up with the epithet "Gay is good." In 1965 he had organized a picket of the White House with signs such as "Sexual preference is irrelevant to federal employment" and "Civil Service is un-American." Yet, confrontational though such a tactic was, the picketers dressed in suits and ties to emphasize their respectability: "Grubbiness has never, to my knowledge, been a stereotype of a homosexual," Kameny insisted.

Other homosexuals prefigured later militant tactics. In New York the remarkable young activist Craig Rodwell had been ahead of his time. In 1964 he thought up an idea that sounds very much like "outing" by suggesting that an ad be placed giving homosexuals five years to reveal themselves: on January 1, 1970, the names of every gay person known would appear. Rodwell had no qualms about stating who he was. When the Alan Burke TV show wanted a "homosexual" to interview, Rodwell jumped at the chance to declare himself. It was Rodwell who founded the Oscar Wilde Memorial Bookshop in Greenwich Village.

In the pre-Stonewall years, San Francisco was the mecca for homosexuals. Eight years before the Stonewall riots the Black Cat bar in San Francisco, which Ginsberg dubbed "the greatest gay bar in America," was a center of resistance when police tried to remove the liquor licenses from twelve of the city's homosexual bars. The historian John D'Emilio has immortalized the drag queen José Sarria who virtually single-handedly raised the consciousness of the patrons by singing "God Save Us Nelly Queens." By 1961 Sarria ran as an openly gay man for the San Francisco Board of Supervisors, polling six thousand votes. He lost, but several new homosexual organizations appeared, notably the Society for Individual Rights (SIR). This organization, along with the Mattachine, the Council on Religion and the Homosexual, and the lesbian Daughters of Bilitis, held a ball on January 1, 1965, to raise funds. The police had promised to stay away but instead photographed and harassed the participants, and arrested some of them. The organizations responded with a news conference furiously accusing the police of "deliberate harassment and bad faith." When the case of those arrested came to court, the judge instructed the jury to declare a "not guilty" verdict even before the defense had a chance to make its case. A groundswell of support for gays swept the city, and the police were forced to abandon their attempts to clamp down on gay bars. The gay community now became a political force in the city. Dianne Feinstein when she became city supervisor in 1969, publicly thanked the homosexual community for helping her to victory.

These early successes for gay rights in the sixties were probably helped by the increasing visibility of gay culture in the media—much of it unfavorable. The *New York Times* in 1963 printed an article headed "Growth of Overt Homosexuality in City Provokes Wide Concerns." The piece contained extensive commentary from anti-gay psychiatrists Irving Bieber and Charles Socarides and a lengthy discussion of the chances of cure. Other articles soon appeared across the country, following the *Times*'s lead.

At the end of the decade, gays became more visible in the movies. *The Boys in the Band* (1970) became the first all-gay film, albeit one offering a depressing picture of sad, frustrated men on the verge of middle age. In literature, James Baldwin's *Another Country* (1962) and Mary McCarthy's *The Group* (1963) included much more positive views of gay characters; as obscenity laws crumbled, Grove Press published *City of Night* by John Rechy in 1963, a brutally honest account of New York City's gay underworld. Rechy's follow-up, *Numbers* (1967), introduced the wild world of promiscuous sex. The gay culture that was increasingly visible was not a monogamous world, barely indistinguishable from respectable heterosexuality; it was a loose, freewheeling morality that challenged mainstream American values.

The tone had been set in the 1960s by two hugely influential American cultural figures, Susan Sontag and Andy Warhol. Sontag, in her 1967 essay "On Camp," dedicated to Oscar Wilde, effectively interpreted gay culture for the American intelligentsia. Camp was a "sensibility" that "converts the serious into the frivolous—these are grave matters." Examples of camp were "Tiffany lamps," "Schoedsack's King Kong," "the old Flash Gordon comics." She explicitly equated "camp taste" with homosexuality: "While it's not true that camp taste *is* homosexual taste, there is no doubt a peculiar affinity and overlap." Sontag may have had in mind the prominence of the pop artist Andy Warhol who by the late sixties had created a coterie of actors "who would do his bidding" in a series of art films. In *Flesh, Trash, and Heat* (1968–1972), Joe Dellesandro appeared as a male hustler, a junkie, and a "bored object of other people's lust." Dellesandro in fact was playing himself. These films, Warhol's most commercially successful, brought this underworld to the public. His other actors, now forgotten, were also quite colorful. Ondine was a "homosexual speed freak." Paul America "once gate-crashed a party and slashed all the guests' coats with a hunting knife." Eric Emerson, having been "ostracized" by everyone, was "found dead on the street a short time later." These were perfect actors for Warhol's films of lowlife and erotic obsession that in their sexual explicitness gained notoriety as they took advantage of liberals' contemporary willingness to put up with anything.

Within a year of Stonewall the respectable and cautious homophile movement was all but dead and buried in the avalanche created by the new wave of militant "gay" organizations. Days after the riots the New York Gay Liberation Front began to hold meetings. Borrowing the militant rhetoric of the student and anti-war movements, the GLF saw itself as a new kind of "gay" movement. It insisted that gays "come out": "Come out of hiding. Identify yourself. Make it clear. Celebrate your sexuality." As Carl Wittman declared in his famous Gay Manifesto, "If we are liberated, we are open with our sexuality. Closet queenery must end. Come out." The GLF also insisted that homosexuals be known as "gay." Unlike the homophiles, the GLF had a theory of gay revolution. It saw gays as oppressed by the American system; gays should resist by creating a strong political culture: "the emergence of homosexual liberation communes is a good start," declared Wittman. "Rural retreats, political action offices, food cooperatives, a free school, unalienating bars and after hours places—they must be developed if we are to have even the shadow of a free territory." In keeping with this program the GLF sponsored an array of coffeehouses and dances wherever it established branches. And, in the tradition of sixties radical movements, it linked itself to every cause of the period, from the anti-war movement to the pro-Third World Movement.

This was too much for some of its members. It might be compulsory to like Oscar Wilde if you were gay, but you did not have to turn on to Che Guevara. In December 1969 a new breakaway organization, the Gay Activists' Alliance, was founded. Led by Jim Owles, Marty Robinson, and Arthur Evans, it aimed to focus on gay issues alone in the civil rights tradition. But this was as far as the resemblance went. The GAA pioneered the "Zap," dramatic confrontations with politicians and the media. It did not last long, but its major role was to focus the disparate post-Stonewall gay movement. An offshoot of the GAA, the National Gay Task Force, in

1973 gave renewed vigor to gay reform, becoming the major homosexual rights organization and promising to adopt "the old homophile and the reformist gay and lesbian liberationist approaches into a new hybrid with broader appeal." State after state now repealed their sodomy laws. Illinois had abolished its old law as early as 1962. Connecticut repealed its law in 1971. But the great symbolic victory for gay rights was Idaho's new Adult Consent Law, which removed "all penalties for private homosexual acts between freely consenting persons sixteen years old and older." This was significant because Idaho had long been seen as a symbol of gay oppression following a notorious 1955 "homosexual witch-hunt." Other states followed suit. On the federal level, gay rights received a major boost in December 1971 when Senator Ted Kennedy announced that were he to be elected president he would "issue an executive order" if "necessary" to ensure "basic rights" for homosexuals.

More progress followed. In April 1972 San Francisco passed an addendum to the city's administrative code guaranteeing the prohibition of "discrimination based on sexual orientation." This was a major victory for gay rights. Thus by the mid-seventies the atmosphere for gays had grown much more friendly. Gay Democratic clubs were formed in many cities, and 25 percent of college campuses had gay groups. In the 1976 presidential primaries, eight of the ten declared Democratic candidates gave support to gay rights. Front-runner and eventual winner Jimmy Carter declared specifically that he opposed "all forms of discrimination against individuals, including discrimination on the basis of sexual orientation."

There were numerous other successes. In 1973 the American Psychiatric Association removed homosexuality from its list of "psychiatric disorders." Dave Kopay, a professional football player, came out. So did Technical Sergeant Leonard Matlovich. When he declared his homosexuality to the air force, he was given an honorable discharge. After a protracted legal battle the appeals court ordered that he be reinstated. By then Matlovich was exhausted and, "desperately short of money, he accepted a payoff from the air force." Yet he had become the first gay celebrity, appearing on the cover of *Time* magazine, while in the summer of 1979 NBC ran *Matlovich vs. the Air Force* the first nonfiction gay rights story ever aired, detailing Matlovich's experience. Meanwhile on the West Coast, the San Francisco Castro became the first gay ghetto, attracting thousands of young men throughout the 1970s. In their wake the gay community there found a voice in Harvey Milk, a former lover of Craig Rodwell, who became a leading figure in the American gay movement. With his feisty charisma and his famous "Hope" speech—"Hope that all will be right. Without hope, not only gays, but the black[s], the seniors, the handicapped . . . will give up"—he became a legend—and, more important, city supervisor of one of America's major cities. With a flourishing gay movement, America's gays now had an opportunity for great progress in promoting the recognition of same-sex love.

Gay liberation had its darker side too. In a 1977 essay the astute and acute Australian observer of the American gay scene Dennis Altman described his disillusionment with recent developments in gay culture. "Having returned to Australia from the United States with a case of hepatitis, a disease seemingly rife in those sections of the country I frequented, I must admit to viewing my four weeks in the States with a somewhat jaundiced eye," he began. "America has run out of energy—the intellectual, cultural, political energy that so excited me five years ago. . . . America has become truly decadent." Altman blamed the "commercial gay world" for this. Not only did many male homosexuals now have the "illusion that oppression is a thing of the past," as they "retreat into hedonism," but this was dangerous for the future. Citing Herbert Marcuse, he suggested that growing "social tolerance" could actually become "repressive" as gays forgot that full "acceptance" was a long way off and became complacent patsies of a system that increasingly exploited them for commercial gain. The gay rebellion against traditional morality had been coopted into the system.

Altman was a rare critic from within the gay community of the manic promiscuity that overtook large parts of the gay world in the 1970s. In 1978 the Kinsey Institute published a study of gay men in the San Francisco area which showed that nearly half the whites and one-third of the blacks claimed to have had more than five hundred sexual partners. As the critic Midge Decter cleverly noted, "To have had fifty lovers would be a wide range of experience, to have had five hundred bespeaks the obliteration of all experience." Plenty of gay commentators thought the same. Larry Kramer wrote in his 1977 novel *Faggots,* a tale of a man determined to find love before he reaches forty, "Of the 2,639,857 faggots in New York City, 2,639,857 think primarily with their cocks." Andrew Holleran's 1978 novel *Dancer from the Dance* brilliantly described the aimlessness of the New York gay scene's obsession with possessing beauty.

Disco music provided a soundtrack for the manic hedonism that for many gay men represented the fruits of liberation. After 1974 this style of dance music crossed over to the mainstream, spreading its mindless 4.4 beat and often camp lyrics throughout America. From George MacCrae's sublimely sensual "Rock Your Baby," a trans-Atlantic No. 1 in the summer of 1974, to Chic's "Good Times" in the summer of 1979, disco reigned supreme. Two huge stars emerged: Donna Summer, whose "Love to Love You Baby" allegedly contained twenty-four simulated orgasms, and Gloria Gaynor, whose "I Will

Survive" caught sublimely the difficulties of forming relationships in the disco environment. Established stars such as Diana Ross, with "Love Hangover," soon joined in the craze.

As gay men danced their way through the seventies they embraced not just promiscuity but tried to extend American sexual boundaries way beyond their previous limits: "We're the first generation to live openly as homosexuals. We have no role models. We have to find new ways to live," declared Randy Shilts. Some men took this all too literally. Sadomasochistic practices established themselves in the gay community. But "S and M" was dangerous: "In 1981, the San Francisco coroner, Dr. Boyd Stephens, warned that he was seeing an 'alarming increase in injuries and death from S and M sex.'" This was San Francisco, but the growing genre of the gay porn magazine increasingly featured articles on sadomasochistic sex. *Blueboy* magazine in September 1976 published a theme issue: "S and M 1976." This featured "a man emasculating himself in a blood-spattered bathtub as well as other photo features emphasizing razor blades, bloodied skulls, and burning matches inserted in a man's urethra." The issue created outrage in the gay community. But in the Mineshaft in New York, this fantasy could become a reality. Here a middle-aged man "got down on all fours, naked except for a dog-collar," to bite his master who would be forced to whip him.

Although most gay men avoided S and M, gay relationships changed significantly from older patterns. The Victorian and age-old man-boy love ceased to be the ideal in the urban centers of gay life. One could choose from a whole smorgasbord of relationship styles, from monogamy between two men the same age to open relationships and erotic experimentation. When the urbane Edmund White, in his 1980 *Travels in Gay America,* wrote about his visit to Kansas City, he mocked the older-style relationship: "The compliant, slightly nelly boy and the dominant, quietly masculine man form the usual couple." To his horror they modeled their relationship on "the heterosexual husband and wife." White, from Ohio, noted approvingly that "On the two coasts and in such sophisticated interior cities as Houston, Denver, Chicago, and Minneapolis, the beau ideal is no longer the 'beautiful boy' of eighteen but the 'hot man of 35.' "

By the 1970s heterosexual boundaries in popular culture seemed to be crumbling. Early in the decade Hollywood films experimented with more and more realistic themes. *Bob and Carol and Ted and Alice* (1969) was about wife-swapping, while *Carnal Knowledge* (1971), about student love, was judged "obscene" by the Georgia Supreme Court. Stanley Kubrick's 1971 film *A Clockwork Orange* perhaps encouraged this sort of reaction. The film featured graphic sexual violence and further helped bring about the demise of the X rating. Upon its release, Kubrick simply could not get it publicized. Equally as notorious was the 1972 film *Deep Throat,* which toyed with oral sex. The X-rated cartoon *Fritz the Cat* (1972) also stirred controversy. But the last major studio production to carry the X rating was Bernardo Bertolucci's *Last Tango in Paris* (1972). Marlon Brando played Paul, a rather confused middle-aged man who is living in Paris when his wife commits suicide. He feels that he has known nothing of his wife when it emerges that she has been having an affair for several years behind his back. Paul meets twenty-year-old Jeanne and within minutes they are having wild, passionate, yet emotionless sexual intercourse. The reaction of moralists to the film was led by none other than President Richard Nixon: "American morality is not to be trifled with. The warped and brutal portrayal of sex in books, plays, magazines and movies, if not halted and reversed could poison the wellsprings of American and Western culture and civilization as a whole."

In reaction to the spread of pornography, the forces of censorship began to rally. President Nixon again joined the debate, declaring that "So long as I am in the White House there will be no relaxation of the national effort to control and eliminate smut from our national life." The Los Angeles Police Department began to crack down on porno movie theatres. In June 1973 the Supreme Court returned to the states the right to establish their own community standards. Justice Warren Burger declared, "It is unconstitutional to read the First Amendment as requiring the people of Maine and Mississippi to accept standards of conduct found tolerable in Las Vegas and New York City." Initially this decision had little impact. A film such as Pier Paolo Pasolini's *Salo, or The 120 Days of Sodom* could still be shown. But there were signs of change as early as 1975 when Warren Beatty made *Shampoo* with its sobering view of the sexual revolution. Here Beatty spoofed his off-screen image as a great lover. This film offended many people with its morally dubious characters and its sexual frankness. But the movie was a serious commentary on the costs of the sexual revolution.

By the late 1970s, as with other areas of the sexual revolution, the movies became the targets of feminists and the emerging New Right. *Looking for Mr. Goodbar* (1977) featured a female teacher of deaf and dumb kids who looks for a suitable mate on the singles scene only to be killed by one of her pickups. Despite its obviously sobering tone, the film was banned in Utah. One critic declared it "the most graphic, brutal and sickening display of exploitation I've ever seen."

Still in all, the movies survived the backlash uncensored. By the turn of the decade Dudley Moore and Bo Derek were starring in *10* (1979), an unabashed celebration of sexual liberation. By 1980 the revolt against Victorian morality in the movies was triumphant.

The hedonism of gay culture and of film in the 1970s was rivaled only by that of rock culture. In the late sixties and early seventies rock musicians concerned themselves primarily with drug-taking, but as casualties mounted, rock music again became sexually daring. As in the 1950s, it was driven by the commercial demands of record companies. But it also drew on the creative talents of educated members of a vibrant Anglo-American youth culture. In 1970 the Kinks returned to the American top ten with their classic song "Lola," a comic tale of a young man's encounter with a transsexual with a "dark brown voice." Soon, only a couple of years after Stonewall, the emerging British star David Bowie declared to an interviewer that he was bisexual. Whatever Bowie's true proclivities, the "gay" image he portrayed worked wonders in drawing attention to his work. His onstage simulation of oral sex and his wearing of "men's dresses" all helped to spread the Bowie word. He soon moved on to other images and new ideas, but in his wake the Anglo-American "glam rock" movement flirted with homosexuality and drag. Bowie produced Mott the Hoople's foppish hit "All the Young Dudes" in 1972, and the straight band discovered that "We became instant queers. Of course we weren't. It was all very funny." Bowie also produced Lou Reed's 1973 album *Transformer* with the classic song "Walk on the Wild Side" that spoofed the crowd around Andy Warhol. Reed's earlier band, the Velvet Underground, had dabbled in gay rock with songs like "I'm Waiting for the Man." But with "Walk" he surpassed himself: this top-forty radio hit included lines like "shaved his legs, and then he was a she" and "giving head."

In the 1970s the rock star became a new model for popular-culture hedonism. Rod Stewart, even more than Mick Jagger, typified this trend. Stewart made a virtue out of being "one of the lads," of being a "playboy." His string of affairs and relationships with beautiful actresses and models such as Britt Ekland and Bebe Buell gained wide publicity, so that by the end of the decade his playboy reputation seemed assured. But

Stewart became a model for heterosexual male liberation also because of the frankness of his songs. His first hit, "Maggie May," described his first sexual encounter: he has recently crudely admitted that the real-life Maggie May he'd "shagged . . . three minutes out, three minutes in." His biggest hit, "Tonight's the Night" (1976), was a song about a man seducing a virgin. For many months top-forty radio was dominated by Stewart's lecherous croak and Ekland's orgasmic cooing. By the end of the decade, however, Stewart had lapsed into dirty-old-man bloat when he parodied his image in the disco song "D'Ya Think I'm Sexy?" Stewart was never obscene, but he was often rude and always honest. Radio had not known his like before.

The Rolling Stones by the 1970s were every bit as popular as in the 1960s, but their world-weariness was by now hopelessly contrived. Their 1971 album *Sticky Fingers* featured a cover by Andy Warhol that featured a real zipper that could be unzipped to reveal underwear and a bulge. The Stones went on to make some fabulous rock in the seventies, but when their albums were less spectacular, such as 1976's tepid *Black and Blue,* they felt it necessary to provoke. So the advertising for this album contained a model bound and gagged, and after protests it had to be withdrawn. By 1978's classic album *Some Girls,* the sexism sounded dated and the S and M of "When the Whip Comes Down" and "Beast of Burden" hopelessly contrived. By then these songs were being willingly played on the radio, any resistance long since dissipated by the Stones' popularity.

For the record companies, the rock stars' main purpose was to sell records. This the performers shamelessly did, whatever image they had to adopt to do it. But as with disco hedonism, there were victims. One fan described her Bowie obsession to Fred and Judy Vermorel in 1976: "I was kinky about the fact he was so thin and he was like a woman. He seemed the per-

fect vehicle for my sexual needs and fulfillment." She went on
to find herself a boyfriend who looked like Bowie: "Just the
fact he could look like Bowie was an amazing achievement in
my books." Bowie, for this fan, "prompted something in me
which I didn't know was actually there—he made it popular
to sleep with men and women and he made it popular to be
extreme—and what's more he made it possible to make it like
that every day." But as the fan grew older she saw through her
obsessions: "I think he should be made aware of how he's influenced people's dress, their manners, their behavior. . . . It's a
terrible thing he did really. He's got a lot to answer for."

Another vital development of the 1970s was the emergence
of black rock stars who rejected the Motown image of supper-
club respectability. Isaac Hayes was the first to break ranks.
According to the rock historian Ken Tucker, "he used love-
making as the elaborate, grandly overstated organizing principle of his music. His gentle, rambling spoken introductions
to many songs were the foreplay, while the repetition of simple melodies and the damp layers of orchestral strings delayed
the climax of any given song until almost past endurance."
Hayes's imitator, Barry White, nearly became an international
superstar in the mid-seventies as he grunted and groaned his
way through several more commercial imitations of the sex
act—"I'm Gonna Love You Just a Little Bit More Baby" and
"[It's Ecstasy] When You Lay Down Next to Me." White, a
huge man, was an unlikely sex symbol. This could not have
been said for Marvin Gaye, a handsome man who after his
classic album of environmental concern, *What's Goin' On?*,
turned to sex and sensuality in a number of frank songs: "Let's
Get It On," "You Sure Love to Ball," and, almost despairing in
its understatedness, "I Want You." In 1976 Gaye admitted that
"Yes LGIO was about sex. I wanted to do a record which
looked at physical love in a much more open and honest way
than I'd been given an opportunity to do." The slinkiest and

sexiest soul man of the seventies was Al Green, whose albums played constantly with the tension he felt between his sexual desires and his religion. Perhaps his best song is "Take Me to the River," where he sings of sexual temptations—"Sixteen candles a-burnin' at my door," yet he wishes to be washed free of sexual sin: "Take me to the river and wash me down." In 1979's "Belle," drawing back from the point of coitus, he sings, "It's you that I want but its Him that I need," and one can feel the tension and strain of coitus interruptus. Green, White, Gaye, and Hayes were hugely commercial stars who sang not just for black but for white girls (and gay boys).

Equally as subversive was the changing image of the black female singer. Most female singers and groups in the 1970s carried on in the tradition of the Supremes, wholesome and well groomed. But Tina Turner's first huge single in 1971, "Proud Mary," announced to Americans a much raunchier black female sexuality. Turner's lascivious vocals again were heard on her hyperfunk 1973 tour de force *Nutbush City Limits* before she reemerged in the 1980s as diva and postfeminist survivor. The great Turner with her long legs was always magnificent, never sleazy. This could not be said for Millie Jackson, whose notoriously frank stage show elicited much comment and whose album *Caught Up* (1973) dealt with the problems posed by infidelity and multiple relationships. Forty-three-year-old Sylvia Robinson scored with *Pillow Talk* (1973), an overt imitation of female orgasm. But strongest of all was Patti LaBelle, whose inestimable 1975 *Lady Marmalade* contained the irresistible hook "Voulez vous coucher avec moi ce soir?"

The disco boom peaked in 1978 with the hugely successful movie *Saturday Night Fever*. John Travolta played Vinnie Manero, a heterosexual version of a gay disco bunny. When Travolta started into the famous strut at the beginning of the film, it was clear that the sexualization of American popular culture that for so long had affected women and gay men had finally begun to change heterosexual men. Travolta's persona was no Brando or Dean: he was almost camp as the disco world created by gay men for gay men took over his life. What the filmmaker Dennis Altman in the 1980s called "the homosexualization of America" had already begun, and the castrato voices of the Bee Gees on the *Saturday Night Fever* soundtrack seemed to confirm it.

The result of all this hedonism was a powerful backlash from the pro-family Christian forces in American society. The Catholic writer Joseph Sobran, in *Human Life Review*, advised that homosexuals should be counseled to prevent them from practicing. Another author, Ellen Wilson, warned that homosexual unions were "antithetical to family life." The response of evangelical Protestants was even more critical. In 1977 the singer Anita Bryant, known best at the time for advertising Florida orange juice, embarked on a "Save Our Children" campaign which succeeded in winning repeal of the Dade County (Florida) gay rights ordinance. Bryant stirred into action the National Association of Evangelicals, which consisted of a number of television evangelists, including the PTL Club, the 700 Club, and the Old Time Gospel Hour. Perhaps the most famous of the anti-gay pastors—Virginia's Jerry Falwell—campaigned in person for Bryant. Falwell believed in the responsibility of the Christian to enact Christian values here on earth. His Liberty Baptist Church in Lynchburg was a veritable moral community whose members tried to live the Christian life: the message of Christ as interpreted by Pastor Falwell. In 1976 Falwell began his "I Love America" rallies from the steps of state capitols throughout the country. At these rallies he attacked pornography, homosexuality, abortion, and the ERA. The following year he began a campaign against homosexuals teaching in public schools. Then, in 1978, he helped defeat a gay rights ordinance in Florida. The forward march of the Christian Right, latter-day carriers of the torch of traditional neo-Victorian values, went on. In 1978 Falwell negotiated with a number of right-wing activists for the formation of three new organizations: the Religious Roundtable, the Christian Voice, and the Moral Majority. By 1980 they had become the basis for a powerful conservative alliance, the New Right, which in Ronald Reagan found an apparently sympathetic presidential candidate. So strong were conservative groups in the Republican party that it seemed they might actually come to dominate it. For sexual liberals and sexual liberationists, the turn of the decade seemed to threaten only clampdown and backlash. Was the party over?

7

"When the Hangover Strikes": Sexual Morality at the Turn of the Century

SUMMER 1981 seemed like the start of a new era in American history. For the arrival of Ronald Reagan in the White House lent reassurance to many Americans that twenty years of domestic instability were ending. Certainly Reagan's success in pushing his economic program through Congress that spring—albeit with the help of an attempted assassin's bullet—seemed to lend credence to a growing American optimism.

On July 3, 1981, the *New York Times* published a story that a rare cancer, Kaposi's Sarcoma, had been found in forty-one homosexual men, many of whom also suffered "severe defects in their immunological systems." The article spurred little interest initially outside the gay and lesbian communities of New York and San Francisco. But the American newspaper of record was reporting the onset of the AIDS crisis, and it was not long before the story became big news.

AIDS was to become the single most important development in the area of sexuality for homosexual men and straight Americans over the next twenty years. Only lesbians largely escaped the wrath of HIV. It worked along with numerous other areas of American culture to *advance* the revolt against Victorian morality. The safe-sex boom helped extend the boundaries of sexual explicitness so as to affect the attitudes and behavior of those ordinary Americans who had so far been uninfluenced by the onslaught of popular culture. It also helped expand the varieties of sexual experience on offer. Yet it also served as a warning against the sexual revolution's encouragement of promiscuity. Thus it helped encourage a sense of frustration and of growing emotional and erotic constraint that was symbolized by the growth of sexual correctness. Together with sophisticated survey evidence of the persistence of conservative habits among many Americans, this made for a confusing mosaic.

Such was the sex saturation of the 1980s that the sixties and seventies seem naive and innocent by comparison. Rock music, in its constant search for novelty and outrage led the way in the continuing revolt as the imperative of commercial gain outweighed regard for traditional mores. Popular music of the early eighties romanticized sexual ambiguity and homoeroticism. While David Bowie in his 1983 smash album *Let's Dance* adopted a new butch image and renounced his earlier claims of bisexuality, other Brits were keener to hint at ambiguity, following his earlier lead. At the 1984 Grammy Awards, Annie Lennox of the Eurythmics adopted full male drag to sing "Sweet Dreams Are Made of This," while Boy George outrageously told the audience via satellite: "Thank you, America. You've got good taste, style, and you know a good drag queen when you see one." Other British rock stars of the time notably lacked George's panache in their homoerotic appeal. A grotesque 1985 *Rolling Stone* cover featured Billy Idol clad only in a couple of belts.

For all its gender bending, the British pop invasion of the mid-1980s was small fry compared to the strength of American rock. Of its four leading figures, only Bruce Springsteen espoused "family values," though even his 1987 album *Tunnel of Love* focused on his divorce. Family values did not concern the other three key figures, Madonna, Prince, and Michael Jackson. Jackson emerged at the height of his powers with his 1982 album *Thriller,* still the biggest seller in history. In retrospect, his 1987 follow-up, *Bad,* prefigures later developments. Jackson's crotch-grabbing in the video to "The Way You Make Me Feel" caused much comment at the time, as did the song, "Dirty Diana." Madonna and Prince, though, caused the most scandal. Like British artists they romanticized the unconventional and the ambiguous. Early in the decade Prince's smuttiness probably delayed his commercial emergence. Albums such as *Dirty Mind* (1980) and songs such as "Jack U Off" were a decade ahead of the times for mass consumption. Prince cleaned up his act for his breakthrough albums, *1999* (1982) and *Purple Rain* (1984). But by *Sign O' the Times* (1987) he was back to his old tricks: the song "If I Was You Girlfriend" hinted at gender ambiguity. One critic noted, "All he apparently wants is to wash his girlfriend's hair, pick out her clothes before they go out and then 'dress her' but we know he likes the look of that lacey stuff himself."

Not even Prince could rival Madonna. She may have started "Like a Virgin." But by the 1985 video for "Open Your Heart," she was playing a peep-show performer trying to lure an eleven-year-old boy. She simulates masturbation in her 1989 video for the song "Express Yourself." No wonder Helen Gurley Brown, 1960s champion of the single girl, lavishly praised her: "she looks fantastic, she's a good actress, and I love her clothes. She also has a great body, which you can actually see some of. I know women who have lovely bosoms, thirty-six-inch bosoms, and you wouldn't even know because they wear turtleneck sweaters. If you have such a lovely body, why not make the most of it?"

Madonna's celebration of liberated sexuality, both in its straight and gay form, did not come to full fruition until the 1990s, but her use of videos as virtual soft porn was one of the most important ways that rock aided moral revolt in the period. The growing popularity of MTV was one of the phenomena of the decade. High school and college students were subjected to a stream of erotic images throughout the day as a sales lure. Allan Bloom in his 1987 best-seller *The Closing of the American Mind* was one of the first to notice: "Picture a thirteen-year-old boy sitting in the living room of his family home doing his math assignment while wearing his Walkman headphones or watching MTV. . . . A pubescent child whose body throbs with orgasmic rhythms; whose feelings are made articulate on hymns to the joys of onanism or the killing of parents; whose ambition is to win fame and wealth in imitating the drag queen who makes music. In short, life is made into a nonstop, commercially prepackaged masturbational fantasy." It is no wonder that in 1985 Tipper Gore, wife of then Senator Al Gore, testified before Congress on the need for warning stickers on albums, which duly appeared shortly afterward.

Hollywood was not to be outdone. With the breakdown of the old studio system, combined with the decline of censorship, directors had greater concern than ever with the bottom line. More sex was the answer. Commenting on "The Year in Movies" in *Rolling Stone* magazine in December 1983, David Rosenthal noted Hollywood's portrayal of sexuality that year: "Sex appeal and stupidity have long been the happiest marriage in Hollywood. Show enough flesh, whistle, and people would always plunk down their money. The problem is that today it's all done so artlessly. The teen fantasies of fifties beach movies may have been stilted and artificial, but at least they left something to the imagination. A generation earlier, when Marlene Dietrich or Clark Gable were up to no good, you could always just imagine what no good was. I don't mean to be prudish, but did America need two (count 'em, two) chances in 1983 to see Richard Gere's private part?"

Rosenthal identified a much more open male sexuality in American films that year. Gere had succeeded Travolta as the leading male star after *American Gigolo* (1980) and *An Officer and a Gentleman* (1982). He flaunted his torso at every opportunity. But younger stars too joined in the rush to expose themselves. Tom Cruise in *Risky Business* (where he played a teenage pimp) and in *All the Right Moves* (both 1983), according to Rosenthal, "managed to flex his biceps and drop his drawers to the twittering delight of the zit-cream set." In *Rumble Fish* (1983), "without looking too closely everyone managed to get a glimpse of Matt Dillon's jockey shorts."

Rosenthal noted that this trend to sexualize the male was "not a far cry from formulaic attempts to make a few bucks by showing a few breasts." And the objectification of women, despite feminist outcries, continued unabated. Most notorious was the work of the director Adrian Lyne, who rose to prominence in 1983 with *Flashdance* and its "tits and buns dance numbers." In 1986, however, he excelled himself with *9½ Weeks,* in which a masochistic woman (Kim Basinger) is forced to grovel for money at her stockbroker boyfriend's feet. Lyne then proceeded to surpass himself with Glenn Close's homicidal career woman in *Fatal Attraction* (1987).

Hollywood undermined traditional morality and the family in other ways during the 1980s. Films presented liberated sexualities, be they straight or gay, favorably. The 1982 film *Making Love* was the first mainstream Hollywood movie to present homosexuality in a positive light. This was threatening to a few, but it is now hard to understand why: the affair between Michael Ontkean and Harry Hamlin was tastefully but tentatively done. Even "family" movies such as *Baby Boom* (1987) and *Look Who's Talking* (1989), while they claimed to celebrate childrearing, all featured single parents. Gere's career turned upward in 1990 with *Pretty Woman* which, remarkable though it was, made Cinderella into a prostitute.

Spike Lee, the leading African-American director, has been accused by the critic Michael Medved of "glamorizing illegitimacy." Lee and other black directors, in *Do the Right Thing* (1989), *Boyz N the Hood* (1991), *Juice* (1992), and *Gladiator* (1992), feature attractive young black males who have fathered babies out of wedlock.

Everywhere in American popular culture sexual boundaries expanded further to include an unprecedented growth of explicitly sexual descriptions. Gore Vidal, who in the forties had introduced homosexuality and in the sixties transexuality, in the eighties produced *Duluth,* a petulant blend of all his pet peeves that included rape, sadomasochism, incest—anything and everything but family values, which Vidal loved to disparage.

If the 1920s youth writers had scandalized by referring to a "kiss," and if the Beats had shocked by dabbling in bisexuality, 1980s youth writers such as Jay McInerney and Brett Easton Ellis were as uninhibited as Vidal. Ellis's debut, *Less Than Zero* (1985), in short, staccato bursts and lewd language attempted to capture the aimlessness of the MTV generation.

Advertising continued to objectify women's bodies. Even the conservative and moralistic Coors family advertised their beer in *Rolling Stone* magazine with a girl in a swimsuit. But such images were everywhere in the 1980s: films were advertised with female stars in ever-skimpier clothing. In 1983 Jessica Lange allowed herself to be photographed by Bert Stein prostrate in prostitute's gear with a flower in her mouth. Ads for Calvin Klein's perfume Obsession featured a bevy of naked women.

There was still stronger stuff. As the author Susan Faludi has noted, "The beaten, bound, or body-gagged woman became a staple of the late 1980s fashion ads and editorial layouts. In the windows of major department stores female mannequins were suddenly being displayed as the battered conquests of leather-clad men and as corpses stuffed in rubbish sacks. In *Vogue,* a fashion lay-out entitled "Hidden Delights" featured one model in a blindfold being pulled along by her corset ties, another woman with trussed legs, and still another with her arms and nude torso restrained in straps." Other fashion magazines used women in straitjackets or choke collars. The masochism got worse: one could see a woman on an ironing board having an iron placed on her genitals; or a woman's legs dangling from a man's fist; or a woman pushed on the floor, her shirt ripped open.

Abuse of women had long been routine. What was newer in the 1980s was the objectification of male bodies. The pumping-iron fad of the early to mid-eighties not only gave Travolta a chance to display his torso in ads for the films *Two of a Kind* (1983) and *Perfect* (1985) but also for a number of male models to emerge as stars. The Soloflex equipment system, in particular, created a number of famous TV commercials, notably those with Scott Madsen. Calvin Klein underwear became famous for a series of ads that bestrode vast billboards and the sides of buses in American cities. An early billboard pictured the Brazilian pole-vaulter Tom Hintnaus lying down in his underwear. One executive noted, "They look as if they really fit." Ads for male perfume also featured perfectly honed torsos.

Meanwhile the women's movement in the eighties did not decline but rather diversified. In the process, two fierce battles raged in the existing women's organizations over pornography and "date rape." The attitude of the women's movement toward the sexual revolution had always been ambivalent: feminists suspected that the sexual revolution was male-defined, and they wanted things women's way. Battles in the seventies between lesbian and straight women had been largely resolved by the 1980s when a major new row erupted over pornography.

This battle was fierce. Andrea Dworkin's lurid 1981 book *Pornography: Men Possessing Women* became a staple of women's studies courses across the nation. In this book she developed Robin Morgan's earlier ideas about the link between pornography and rape. Pornography, Dworkin argued, was the major way by which men kept women down: "The woman's sex is appropriated, her body is possessed, she is used and she is despised: the pornography does it and the pornography proves it." Dworkin went so far as to see the penis as a "symbol of terror." Together with the lawyer Catharine MacKinnon, she worked on an ordinance to ban pornography in Minneapolis and then Indianapolis. Because of the support the ordinances received from the Christian right, Dworkin has often been accused of supporting a return to Victorianism because, once again, women are expected to check what the philosopher Roger Scruton has called "the unbridled ambition of the phallus." But Dworkin and MacKinnon's real target was heterosexual sex. As such, their rebellion was against nature itself.

This was reflected too in the concern over date rape, which had been prefigured in Dworkin and MacKinnon's 1980s efforts to stamp out porn and in their suspicion of heterosexuality. A 1985 *Ms.* magazine survey conducted by Mary Koss, "The Date Rape Epidemic and Those Who Denied It," claimed that no less than one in four college women had experienced rape or attempted rape. Following the much-publicized trial for date rape of William Kennedy Smith in 1991, the issue became the focus of heated public debate, especially on university campuses which for years had been pouring money into warning women of the dangers of rape. Men got warnings too: the pioneering 1983 Ohio State University Men's Curriculum Task Force Against Rape set up a team of idealistic young men to go into the dorms and try to teach undergraduate men about appropriate behavior: with the ultimate worthy goal of ending all rape. But the problem of rape, alas, did not go away; its intransigence by the 1990s led to far more dramatic measures. As the jurist Robert Bork has explained it, "The eagerness of radical feminists to see insult in every male action, coupled (if one dare use that word) with the spinelessness of the patriarchy, has led to so much discomfort and loss of freedom." Hence at the University of Pennsylvania a young man who told a young woman that she had "nice legs" was accused of committing a "mini rape." At the University of Maryland female students posted the names of male students entirely at random, claiming they were all "potential rapists."

These young women were merely echoing the pamphlets they had been given by the university administration or the rhetoric they had learned in women's studies classes. Students read Susan Brownmiller's *Against Our Will* and Andrea Dworkin's work. They read Brownmiller's famous remark that "Since you may not know who has the potential for rape, be on your guard with every man . . . the typical American rapist might be the boy next door." One typical pamphlet that followed the party line was entitled "Is Dating Dangerous?" Another advised young women to "think carefully before you go to a male friend's apartment or dorm. . . . Do not expose yourself to unnecessary risk." Students saw, horrified, the HBO drama about date rape, *The Katie Koestner Story,* a tale of a virgin who, touchingly, still slept with a stuffed animal, yet who was forced to have sex.

Antioch College in Yellow Springs, Ohio, a small, expensive liberal arts college, took feminist rape analysis the most seriously. Antioch's thirteen-page Sexual Offense Prevention Policy set up a veritable "dictatorship of virtue": "The person who initiates sexual behavior is responsible for verbally asking for the consent of the other individual(s) involved." But consent wasn't enough; it had to be communicated and recommunicated again and again. At any point the lover could say "no." Then the other individual had to stop immediately. Would-be lovers were told that they should obtain consent for each new physical stage in the relationship—holding hands, touching, kissing, and making love.

The Antioch code and other excesses upset many writers. Katie Roiphe, in her 1993 polemic against the date-rape industry *The Morning After,* sensed a creeping Victorianism on campuses. But this was not Victorianism; quite the opposite. Rather it was a response to the collapse of Victorian morality. The historian Elizabeth Fox-Genovese noted in *Feminism Without Illusions* (1991) that "Although the sexual revolution has 'liberated' young women from many of the older constraints of propriety, it has also deprived them of the attendant protections. . . . [They] have cause to worry that when they choose not to have sexual relations with a particular man their 'no' might not be respected. The ensuing confusion has given rise to the epidemic of 'acquaintance rape' on campuses." Of course, had colleges like Antioch kept their earlier stringent policies of separating the sexes in a Victorian manner, such concerns and suspicions might not have been necessary. But it was too late to turn back the clock. The new code was here to stay, and it revealed the contradictions in America's post–sexual-revolution mood—on the one hand, sexuality should be expressed; on the other, the other gender should be regarded with suspicion. The sexual revolution had not liberated these college students; it had frustrated them.

The struggles in the women's movement over pornography and date rape were of some cultural significance. But they paled in comparison with the AIDS crisis. At first, and notoriously, the story grew only within the gay community: the first TV special on AIDS appeared only in August 1982. In that year the *New York Times* published five stories on the epidemic. By then the gay community had begun to push the issue. On January 4, 1982, Edmund White and Larry Kramer, among others, founded the Gay Men's Health Crisis, which aimed to help AIDS-stricken New Yorkers. Kramer's call-to-arms in a March 1983 edition of the *New York Native*, "1112 and Counting," is a classic indictment of the smug, self-satisfied, and ostrich-like failure of gay and straight Americans to rally round to resolve the crisis: "I am sick of everyone in this community who tells me to stop creating a panic. How many of us have to die before you get scared off your ass into action? Aren't 195 dead New Yorkers enough? Every straight person who is knowledgeable about the AIDS epidemic can't understand why gay men aren't marching on the White House.... I am sick of guys who moan that giving up careless sex until this blows over is worse than death.... Come with me guys while I visit a few of our friends in intensive care at NYU. They'd give up sex forever if you could promise them life."

In 1984, when the virus was discovered and a test developed to determine its presence, the full extent to which the disease had infiltrated the gay community became known as thousands of gay men throughout the country went to physicians or clinics to discover their fate: a positive result in those days meant death. One night in Columbus, Ohio, in December 1985 everyone that went to be tested at the city's major clinic was positive: an eerie chill swept over the heartland.

Needless to say, people such as Kramer and other gay leaders knew that this crisis would make or break the gay community. At first they found an unwillingness to publicize AIDS. Checks on sexual expression were deeply sensitive to gays who believed their newly won freedoms were about to be rolled back.

Far from halting the spread of promiscuity that had been a key development of the sexual revolution in the gay community, the emergent AIDS bureaucracy had a stroke of genius:

the safer-sex industry. Safer sex, a direct consequence of the AIDS crisis, did perhaps more than anything else—even Madonna—in the 1980s to extend the revolt against Victorian morality. For the irony of the AIDS crisis was that the AIDS bureaucracy saw its solution not as abstinence but as more "sex"—if "sex" were "safe."

By the late eighties it was hard to avoid the endless stream of pamphlets that advocated safer sex, informing an ever-broader population of the different alternatives to unsafe sex. Ordinary Americans found out about oral sex and anal sex; and the pamphlets often used crude language such as "fucking" and "sucking." Above all, the safer-sex industry stressed the use of condoms. What had previously been seen as a moderately effective form of birth control now became the key that opened the door to ever-safer sex.

Safer sex neatly encapsulated the dilemma that Americans now faced. The safer-sex industry was, on the one hand, a massive government-sponsored attempt to expand sexual boundaries and to continue the sexual revolution. On the other hand, it was a great dampener of passions: for many people, condoms spoiled the party. Safer sex merely added to the sex saturation that pervaded American culture in the 1980s. But it also provoked the frustration of unfulfilled, ever-growing expectations.

Not only did the stress on condom use continue the divorce of sexuality from reproduction that had been developing throughout the twentieth century, it also removed fundamental aspects of the enjoyment of the act. As one psychologist has noted, "The unmentionable aspect of wearing a condom is that it isn't just *physical* sensitivity that is affected, but emotional sensitivity as well. There is something about the contact with naked flesh that provides a unique physical and emotional 'connectedness.'" Not only this, but safer sex aimed to prevent the mixing of bodily fluids by ensuring that a piece of rubber latex be placed in the way. Yet the process threatened to reduce intimacy between men and women and men and men, and to inhibit love itself. In the gay community, for example, a vogue for "safer-sex" erotic stories arose. One such story even advocated "navel fucking."

How much sex were Americans now having? Since Kinsey and Masters and Johnson, it had been assumed that Americans were as freewheeling and liberated as the constant "sex on display" in American society suggested. But Kinsey's methodology still raised doubts, and Masters and Johnson seemed dubious. Shere Hite *was* dubious. In 1994, a team of sociologists headed by Robert T. Michael published *Sex in America: A Definitive Survey,* a work that attempted to use state-of-the-art sociological techniques in an effort to update Kinsey but also to gauge what American behavior was like in a land of sex saturation. The results stunned many. They confirmed that Americans remained deeply conservative in their behavior, and that popular culture, the site of so much of the revolt against Victorian sexual morality, was not a true reflection of what Americans practiced. The authors eventually went so far as to claim that there had not been a sexual revolution because the average number of sexual partners that Americans had over their life course had not significantly increased. About a third of Americans aged over fifty had had five or more partners in their lifetime; half of all Americans aged thirty to fifty had had five or more partners. This did not suggest a huge difference. Further, most Americans, when asked about the number of partners that they had had over the last year, answered zero or one. This was scarcely bacchanalian. Equally the authors stressed the ongoing importance of marriage as an institution: "Marriage is such a powerful social institution that, essentially, married people are nearly all alike—they are faithful to their partners as long as the marriage is intact."

The persistence of conservative attitudes and behavior among Americans was confirmed too by the surprisingly low figure for homosexuality, at least compared to Kinsey. About 2.7 percent of the men in the sample had had sex with a man in the last twelve months; while about 4 percent had had such sex with a man over the past five years, and 5 percent since age eighteen. Nine percent of men had had sex with a man since puberty. About 5 percent admitted attraction to a person of the same gender while 3 percent self-identified as gay. These figures for men were much smaller than Kinsey's famous findings of 37 percent having had sex since puberty and 10 percent over the previous three years. The new figures suggested that a relatively small minority was having great influence and impact on the appearance of American morality through overrepresentation of homosexuality in the media and the arts. The survey confirmed the persistence of older patterns and a real resistance to change. Attitudes towards sexual morality by the 1990s showed the continuing power of Victorianism despite the assault by popular culture. Thus 33.6 percent of Americans believed "there should be laws against the sale of pornography to adults." Just over 76 percent continued to believe that "extramarital sex is always wrong," and 64.8 percent that "same gender sex is always wrong." Ultimately the Victorian romantic ideal remained powerful: 65.7 percent of Americans insisted they "would not have sex with someone unless [I] was in love with them," while 52.3 percent claimed to have been guided by religious beliefs in their sexual behavior.

On the other hand, the study did turn up significant changes in sexual morality. The authors noted a widespread acceptance of sex before marriage. Only 19.7 percent of Americans believed that "premarital sex is always wrong." (A 1994 study by Lilian Rubin found the working class less disposed toward premarital sex than the middle class was.) There had also been a declining age for teenage first intercourse. Those born between 1933 and 1942 averaged first sex at about eighteen. Those born in the sixties first had sex when they were about six months younger. Further, the percentage of women who were virgins at twenty or who had had only one partner had fallen from 84 percent among those born between 1933 and 1942 to 50 percent among those born after 1953. Intriguingly, the percentage of men who were virgins at twenty had actually been rising. This probably reflected the decline of prostitution as an institution.

A second pattern emerged with the sexual revolution: cohabitation. Among those born in the years 1933 to 1942, 84.5 percent of the men and 93.8 percent of the women had married without having lived with a partner beforehand. Of the men born in the years 1963 to 1974, only 33 percent married without cohabiting, and 35.3 percent of the women did. The survey failed to examine another phenomena that had been stirring up controversy too: illegitimacy. The sociologist Charles Murray, in provocative works in the 1980s and 1990s, noted its prevalence in African-American communities. But the problem went beyond African Americans: fatherlessness was widespread. In 1960 the percentage of all American children living with mothers only was 7.7 percent; by 1990 the figure was 21.6 percent. Significantly, 31.5 percent of these children lived with mothers who had never married. In the past, of course, fatherlessness had been common as a result of death. Now it was common because of abandonment. As David Blankenhorn has noted, "For the first time in the nation's history, millions of men today are voluntarily abdicating their fatherhood." Charles Murray noted the effect on children: they would "run wild" with "a level of physical unruliness which makes life difficult."

Michael also noted the ongoing popularity of divorce. Those born between 1933 and 1942 had a four in five chance of their marriages lasting ten years. But among those born between 1953 and 1962, the chance was only three in five. The historian Tamara Hareven explained to a congressional committee that "Divorce now has a similar effect on family disruption that death once had."

The spread of alternative sexual practices would have horrified Victorians. This was particularly true of oral sex. Marriage manuals of the 1920s had referred to "the genital kiss," which was not meant to be a sexual practice at all but rather a means of expressing affection. But since the 1960s oral sex had become popular. Among men aged eighteen to forty-four, half indicated that "receiving oral sex" was "very appealing"; "giving oral sex" was "very appealing" to 37 percent. Among older respondents, those aged forty-five to fifty-nine, receiving oral sex appealed to only 29 percent, while "giving oral sex" appealed to only 22 percent. As the authors themselves noted, "Much larger percentages of women under age fifty as compared to those over fifty have given or received oral sex in their lifetimes. And those in the oldest age group were less than half as likely to have had or received oral sex the last time they had sex. This is suggestive evidence that oral sex came into vogue in the 1960s."

Here, then, was a highly charged situation: a culture saturated in sex yet with deeply contradictory views about it when it came to real attitudes and behavior. The society revealed persistent Victorianism, on the one hand, and, on the other, the growing influence of the sexual revolution. Men and women, however, had very different experiences. Men, in general, were highly sexually active. Between the ages of eighteen and twenty-four, only 15 percent had not had intercourse in the previous six months. Men in their thirties were most sexually active once relationships had been established. Men in fact continued to have fairly regular sex into their sixties. For women, the period of most frequent sex was their forties; but

30 percent of women aged fifty to fifty-nine did not have sex at all compared to 11 percent of men. The sociologist Laurel Richardson, in an influential 1986 book, *The New Other Woman,* noted the desperation of some women who were driven to affairs with married men—who refused to divorce their wives in order to marry their lovers. This strikingly different gender experience was confirmed too by the alarming percentage of women who believed they had been *forced* to have sex. Twenty-two percent of all women thought they had at some stage been forced. Thus a further aspect of the revolt against Victorian morality was the different experiences of men and women. Women apparently had not benefitted as much as men from the sexual revolution.

Another sign of the breakdown of consensus on sexual behavior was the growth of the so-called men's movement, a nineties reaction against the radical feminist movement. As one man put it, "I knew that men had done bad things— started wars, polluted the environment, discriminated against women and all that. But I was tired of hearing from feminists that all men were rotten to the core. There's a lot of good in men."

The 1991 best-seller *Iron John* by Robert Bly brought the movement to national visibility. Across the land men went on retreats with one another in an effort to uncover "the wild man within" that feminists had supposedly stifled. They tried to rediscover a sense of continuity with their fathers. Bly believed "that men suffer because they are cut off from their feelings; that meeting work and family obligations is not enough to keep men spiritually alive; that men need a chance to play like male animals with other men; that feminist criticism of men and masculinity has caused many men to suffer a crisis of confidence; and that men need to be initiated into a secure sense of manhood." Although he rejected feminist analysis, he was not explicitly anti-feminist. He blamed industrialization: "The death of the sacred King and Queen means that we live now in a system of industrial domination, which is not patriarchy. The system we live in gives no honor to the male mode of feeling." Following Bly's lead, thousands of American men became "weekend warriors," gathering at camps throughout the country to rediscover their relationship with nature, and with one another, that had disappeared with Victorian romantic friendship. As the sociologist Michael Kimmel has astutely put it, these men "tap into a deep current of malaise among American men."

At the same time there was evidence of a "shift to moderation" among lesbians. They benefitted from the expansion of women's careers, which created a safe lesbian bourgeoisie comfortably cocooned in the suburbs. Even middle-class lesbianism, because it was explicitly sexual, differed from Victorian "romantic friendship," but many of these women acted and behaved much like their Victorian counterparts in the "female world of love and ritual" had done.

For gay men the 1990s brought new identities. With the development of various drug cocktails that prolonged life, AIDS became less of a primary issue. Yet the gay movement benefitted from the revitalization prompted by the AIDS crisis. The zapping tactics of the gay activist group Act Up in the late 1980s stirred a radicalism into the movement that had not been present since Stonewall. Queer Nation emerged in New York in the spring of 1990 and soon influenced the whole gay movement. Its in-your-face tactics involved kiss-ins in shopping malls and straight bars, but it also shifted the intellectual focus of homoerotic politics. Gays now became "queers," who included all the sexually disfranchised among their ranks—homosexuals, bisexuals, transgendered, and even sympathetic straights. As the gay studies sociologist Barry Adam has shown, queer theory self-consciously broke from the past: "Its claim to an identity that is more inclusive than gay or lesbian inevitably stumbled over a series of oppositions and exclu-sions. Neither historical (such as romantic friendships) nor an-thropological forms of same-sex bonding have any connection to the 'queer.' . . ." But most gays still preferred the tried and tested "gay" identity, which now became a force for conser-vatism: one 1993 best-seller demanded *A Place at the Table* for gays—entry into the American mainstream. By the mid-nineties the question of gay marriage was widely debated. In an impassioned 1995 polemic, *Virtually Normal,* the journalist Andrew Sullivan (himself gay) argued that gay marriage was the fundamental way for gays to integrate: "Gay marriage is not a radical step, it is a profoundly humanizing, traditionaliz-ing step. It is the first step in any resolution of the homosexual question—more than any other institution, since it is the most central institution to the nature of the problem, which is to say, the emotional and sexual bond between one human being and another. If nothing else were done at all, and homosexual marriage were legalized, ninety percent of the political work necessary to achieve homosexual and lesbian equality would have been achieved. It is ultimately the only reform that truly matters."

Although Americans continued to be remarkably conserva-tive in their behavior, the relentless promotion of sexuality and sexual transgression continued unabated in popular culture. In the 1990s, as in the 1980s, Madonna played a role. Her 1992 soft-porn book *Sex* was a calculatingly outrageous attention-seeker designed to disguise her (temporary) loss of musical in-spiration. Her 1993 film *Truth or Dare* exhibited her raunchy way of life: when her father indicates he feels uncomfortable with her taking her clothes off, she tells him she has to con-sider her "art." Her 1995 smash single "Secret" is about a lover whom she discovers masturbates.

Prince too continued his influence with his 1991 album *Di-amonds and Pearls.* Of its two lead singles, one was an injunction to "Gett Off," the other, "Cream," was an ode to semen to the tune of "96 Tears." But Prince could not compete with the popularity of gangsta rap, one of the popular-culture phenomena of the decade. Gangsta rap's sexual explicitness in songs like "Pretty Tied Up" and "Horny" took rock farther than ever before along the path of sexual rebellion.

In mid-decade the British—and women—struck again in the guise of the Spice Girls. Originally five girls, the group specialized in an upfront watered-down version of what Madonna had been doing in the 1980s. The Girls deliberately leaked enticing details of their lives before they had joined together—their nude modeling, their former boyfriends—in an effort to boost their risqué image. As ever, the record industry celebrated nontraditional moralities.

Hollywood continued its sexual objectification of women as before. Two actresses, Sharon Stone and Demi Moore, were close to porn stars in their style. Sharon Stone became a superstar overnight when she crossed her legs in the 1992 film *Basic Instinct.* She went on to some rather less seductive roles. Not so Demi Moore, whom interviewer Dennis Pennis once asked, "Are we ever going to see you in a film in which you keep your clothes on?" This seemed too much to ask. In *Indecent Proposal* (1993) she slept with Robert Redford for a million dollars. In *Disclosure* (1994) she played a woman who charged Michael Douglas with sexual harassment; the film was advertised by billboards that revealed Moore in flagrante delicto. In *Striptease* (1996) she perhaps went too far for her audience, playing a woman who turns to stripping in order to pay the rent.

The major American television networks, which had encouraged the wholesome apple-pie family values of *Leave It to Beaver* and *Ozzie and Harriet* in the 1950s, and *The Waltons* as late as the 1970s, was driven to expand sexual boundaries by its ratings war with cable. For example, in the 1991–1992 season on *Beverly Hills 90210*, seventeen-year-old Brenda lost her virginity to Dylan. Roseanne took her sixteen-year-old daughter to the gynecologist to get some birth-control pills, only to discover that she was already having sex. As Dougie Howser reached eighteen, he went to bed with a woman for the first time: "Being a virgin is driving me nuts." Vice President Dan Quayle in September 1992 railed at the morality of the sitcom *Murphy Brown*. Murphy, a TV newswoman, had by her former husband a child whom she decided to raise alone. Quayle declared: "It doesn't help much when prime-time TV has Murphy Brown . . . bearing a child alone and calling it another 'lifestyle choice.'" Later in the decade, Rosanne attempted to boost her flagging ratings by having a lesbian kiss her on her show. And in 1997 Ellen DeGeneres famously came out on her sitcom. This was meant to horrify Middle America, but instead this calculated ploy to boost ratings bored them, and the show was soon dropped by the network.

The increasing sexual explictness of sitcoms was as nothing by comparison with the talk shows. Phil Donahue had pioneered talk-show frankness with interviews that introduced the nation to gays, feminists, and the like in the 1970s. By the 1980s Oprah Winfrey was doing so even more successfully. But lesser figures such as Sally Jesse Raphael and Montel Williams showed little discretion in what they were prepared to discuss. One Williams show, for example, discussed shore parties: how people took holidays and indulged in sex with multiple partners, tallying the score on bits of paper on the refrigerator door. Another show featured women who married their rapists.

Popular culture had challenged boundaries before, but the 1990s brought public and televised sex scandals. In 1988 presidential candidate Gary Hart had been forced to drop out of the race for the Democratic nomination when photographed on the yacht *Monkey Business* with Donna Rice, with whom he was having an extramarital affair. This scandal was just the beginning. The 1991 hearings for the nomination to the Supreme Court of Clarence Thomas sadly set the tone for the decade. When a former assistant, Anita Hill, accused Thomas of sexual harassment, a nation gasped at the explicitness of the claims in the televised hearings. Tales of Coca-Cola cans entered the nation's living rooms and folklore. When Lorena Bobbitt cut off her husband's penis, many feminists found great amusement. In 1993 scandal erupted around Michael Jackson when a thirteen-year-old accused him of sexual harassment. The case dragged on for the best part of a year as the specter of child abuse raised its head. Even after the Jackson story faded from the headlines, concerns over child sexual abuse continued to grow. Repressed-memory syndrome (now largely discredited) involved thousands of people imagining that their parents had abused them as children. Yet in some surveys over a third of women claim to have been victims of childhood abuse, defined as "unwanted sexual touching." This raised the unwholesome specter of incest too, which elicited a great deal of discussion. David Finkelhorn proposed an alarming link between incest and child abuse rates and changing gender relations: "Men who are comfortable relating to women at the same level of maturity and competence will be less likely to exploit children sexually. As men's relations with women change, so will their relations with children." The specialness of sex that Victorians had so carefully tried to guard in the private world was well and truly spoiled by the pervasiveness of such discussion in the public world.

The excesses of the popular culture continue to spark a vigorous counterattack in defense of traditional morality. Phyllis Schlafly in November 1997 railed at "Academia's War on Marriage" in her *Eagle Forum* newsletter. In this piece the veteran conservative activist attacked an article which had appeared in the *Radcliffe Quarterly* that argued: "Instead of getting married for life, men and women (in whatever combination suits their sexual orientation) should sign up for a 'Seven-Year Hitch' only." She railed at a feminist who described divorce as "a significant life event that confronts individuals with the opportunity to change." Schlafly described her *Eagle Forum*'s mission "to enable conservative and pro-family men and women to participate in the process of self-government and public policy making so that America will continue to be a land of individual liberty, with respect for family integrity, public and private virtue, and private enterprise."

Another example of the continued strength of supporters of family and traditional values was the emergence in the mid-1990s of the Promise Keepers. This organization mobilized Christian men for an enormous march on Washington that emphasized "practicing spiritual, moral, ethical, and sexual purity" and "building strong marriages and families, through love, protection and biblical values"—in other words, the men tried to practice all the classic Victorian virtues. By 1996, 1.1 million men had participated in events at twenty-two stadiums across the country, and the organization had achieved an annual revenue of $87 million.

Another call for a return to Victorianism came from the journalist Wendy Shalit. In her *A Return to Modesty: Discovering the Lost Virtue* (1999), she criticized the sex saturation of modern American society: "Our obsession with sex is to blame for anorexia, depression, stalking and rape." She criticized sex education, the Pill, and even coed dorms. Above all, though, she objected that modesty was no longer seen as a positive characteristic in women at century's end. Shalit, like the Victorians, understood the erotic power of modesty. Nor was she alone. Many high school girls signed pledges to remain virgins until marriage, and other writers sought a return to older systems of etiquette, believing, as the Victorians had, that strong rules in social relations gave women power.

Equally as important during the nineties was a shift in the focus of sex education toward abstinence. In 1999, surveys by the Alan Guttmacher Institute and the Kaiser Family Foundation found that most school districts had shifted their approach to sex education over the previous ten years: a third now placed more emphasis on abstinence from sex. In part this reflected the growing national influence of the conservative South. By 1999, 55 percent of Southern school districts had adopted sex education that stressed abstinence, compared to only 20 percent in the North. This change was greatly accelerated by 1996 legislation that allocated $440 million in state and federal funds to abstinence-only policies. Also in 1999, Republican presidential contender and Texas governor George W. Bush called for "federal spending on an abstinence message equal [to] the $135 million a year now supporting education on contraception." Meanwhile Governor Jeb Bush of Florida set aside $10 million toward abstinence-only sex education in his state. Thus in the 1990s sex education, long at the heart of the revolt against Victorian morality, found itself more and more challenged.

If century's end saw a marked but nostalgic yearning for older certainties, the sex scandals involving President Bill Clinton were the most dramatic yet. Sex had been Clinton's Achilles' heel from the outset of his political career. In 1993, on becoming president, almost his first act was an attempt to permit gays in the military, which led to a serious clash with the military establishment. But Clinton's largest problem involved his own heterosexual proclivities. During his 1992 presidential campaign he had been accused of having a lengthy affair with a woman named Gennifer Flowers. In a carefully staged joint interview, future First Lady Hillary

Rodham Clinton declared the solidity of her marriage, thereby saving her husband's campaign. But rumors about Clinton persisted: a group of Arkansas state troopers claimed they had been hired to get women for him while he was governor. A woman named Paula Jones stated that in 1991 Governor Clinton had exposed himself to her in a hotel room. Most serious of all, however, were the admissions of former White House intern, Monica Lewinsky, that she had engaged in a sexual relationship with the president. Clinton denied this in an address to the American people and under oath to a grand jury. Then, seven months later, he admitted he had lied, but that legally he had told the truth because of the nature of the sexual relationship. Speculation abounded as to what they had actually done until a report by special counsel Kenneth Starr revealed graphic details. The lack of outrage that most Americans felt at the details of the report, and the continuing popularity of the president, illustrated the extent to which Americans had been desensitized by the twentieth-century revolt against traditional morality. Perversely, the subsequent impeachment and the trial of the president dramatically demonstrated how far the personal had come to dominate the politics of 1990s America. The strict split between the public and private worlds that the Victorians had made central to their society had now been reversed; the line between public and private had been collapsed.

Although Clinton was widely regarded as having an excessive sex drive, as suffering from a "sex addiction," his experience was not untypical of his generation. Sex had become a release from the intense effort that his life required. Clinton practiced the sexual acts that his generation had made popular, but he remained unsatisfied. Other men of his age clearly felt much the same—without of course wishing to imitate the president's extremes—as the rush to take Viagra among those who lacked Clinton's potency showed.

By the turn of the millennium it was impossible to escape the discussion of intimate acts, even in one's living room. And the situation is unlikely to change. By the mid-nineties the Internet saw to that. The critic Simon Winchester called it "an untramelled, uncontrolled, wholly liberated ocean of information." Sadly, the Internet rapidly became a pornographer's paradise. One web site featured stories of child castration and rape, including pictures of sex with animals and naked children, not to mention incest. And the Internet was hard to control. The practice of "talking dirty" on the Internet became almost as popular as the craze for telephone sex. Many Americans had abandoned the Victorians' loving sex aimed at procreation in favor of the "virtual sex" that technology had to offer.

American society had been sold out—for commercial gain—to sexual diversity, variety, and thrills. The twentieth-century revolt against Victorian sexual morality dared to promise liberation without commitment. But it failed to deliver. Not only had the behavior and attitudes of most Americans recognized the excesses of popular culture, but the forces of traditional morality, in all their different guises, always resurfaced after each attack. They remained strong. As Americans entered a new millennium, jaded from their experiences of the 1990s, they could anticipate further battles over sexuality. A new generation, rekindling its dream of a better world, might well draw upon the wisdom and common sense of its Victorian great-grandparents.

A Note on Sources

THE MODERN HISTORY of sexuality begins with Michel Foucault, *The History of Sexuality* (3 vols.) (New York, 1976). This is less a history than a rather grandiose and pretentious philosophical speculation on the meaning of sex in the late twentieth century. Reading between the lines, one detects a massive attempt by one man to come to terms with his homosexuality. In United States history the major work is John D'Emilio and Estelle Freedman, *Intimate Matters: A History of Sexuality in America* (New York, 1988), a work meant as a spur to further work—but it is so good it threatens to overwhelm the field. But do not underestimate an earlier work: Sydney Ditzion, *Marriage, Morals, and Sex in America* (New York, 1953), which remains pertinent and relevant. A neglected theoretical work is Roger Scruton, *Sexual Desire: A Philosophical Investigation* (London, 1986).

Much of the most compelling work on sexuality has been on homosexuality. George Chauncey, Jr., *Gay New York: Gender, Urban Culture, and the Making of the Gay Male World, 1890–1940* (New York, 1994) is the first half of a projected history that will take us up to the Stonewall riots. It is one of the finest works in recent American social history. Neil Miller, *Out of the Past: Gay and Lesbian History from 1869 to the Present* (New York, 1995), while focused on the United States, is international in scope. Barry Adam, *The Rise of a Gay and Lesbian Movement* (Boston, 1995) is more political in focus. Lesbianism has been fortunate in two histories: Lillian Faderman, *Odd Girls and Twilight Lovers: A History of Lesbian Life in Twentieth-Century America* (New York, 1991), and Elizabeth Kennedy and Madeline Davis, *Boots of Leather, Slippers of Gold: The History of a Lesbian Community* (New York, 1993).

There is a need for a large general survey on heterosexuality. Meanwhile we have Jonathan Ned Katz, *The Invention of Het-*

erosexuality (New York, 1995). There is a substantial body of work on the history of the family; the most satisfactory recent survey is Steven Mintz and Susan Kellogg, *Domestic Revolutions: A Social History of American Family Life* (New York, 1988). Steven Seidman has attempted two ambitious surveys: *Romantic Longings* (New York, 1991) and *Embattled Eros* (New York, 1992), which argue that a clash between romance and liberation has colored gender relations in the twentieth century. Another work with a compelling thesis and with much material on sexuality is James Lincoln Collier, *The Rise of Selfishness in America* (New York, 1993). Equally as "controversial" is the chapter on sexuality in John Burnham, *Bad Habits: Drinking, Smoking, Taking Drugs, Gambling, Sexual Misbehavior, and Swearing in American History* (New York, 1993). Rochelle Gurstein, *The Repeal of Reticence* (New York, 1996) is a history of censorship that argues that liberalization has caused Americans to exchange intense privacy for less intense intimacy. Francesca Cancian, *Love in America* (New York, 1987) sees intimacy in much more positive terms.

American women's history has numerous surveys. The best for sexuality (and the best in general) is Sara Evans, *Born for Liberty: A History of Women in America* (New York, 1988). But the British pioneer in the field, Sheila Rowbotham's *A Century of Women: The History of Women in Britain and the United States in the Twentieth Century* (New York, 1997) offers an invaluable cross-cultural perspective. There is growing recognition that men have a history too. Michael Kimmel's *Manhood in America* (New York, 1996) is an excellent early attempt to fill the gap. But Peter Filene's *Him/Her/Self: Gender Identities in Modern America* (3rd ed., Baltimore, 1998) has proven remarkably durable.

Among edited collections on sexuality, George Chauncey, Jr., Martin Duberman, and Martha Vicinus, eds., *Hidden from History* (New York, 1989) is international in scope. Kathy Peiss and Christina Simmons, eds., *Passion and Power: Sexuality in History* (Philadelphia, 1989) is the best collection in American history. Also good is Barbara Melosh, ed., *Gender and American History Since 1890* (New York, 1993).

Works that focus on specific aspects of gender and sexual history include Glenda Riley, *Divorce: An American Tradition* (New York, 1991), a celebration of marital breakdown. There are two very different surveys of courtship. Beth Bailey, *From Front Porch to Back Seat: Courtship in Twentieth-Century America* (Baltimore, 1988) is a clever if under-researched qualitative introduction. John Modell's quantitative survey, *Into One's Own: From Youth to Adulthood in the United States* (Berkeley, 1989), is invaluable.

An early history of abortion was James C. Mohr, *Abortion in America* (New York, 1975). See also Leslie Reagan, *When Abortion Was a Crime* (Berkeley, 1997) for an important update from a feminist perspective. The best history of birth control is James Reed, *From Private Vice to Public Virtue* (New York, 1978). See also Linda Gordon's *Women's Body, Women's Right* (New York, 1976), a product of a peculiarly 1970s perspective that men had nothing to do with reproduction. A recent work is Elizabeth Siegel Watkins, *On the Pill: A Social History of Oral Contraceptives, 1950–1970* (Baltimore, 1997).

VICTORIAN MORALITY

The idea that Victorians were repressed about sex has been called by Michel Foucault "the repressive hypothesis." One of Foucault's goals was to expose this idea as a fallacy. But the "repressive hypothesis" has retained great influence in American history. See especially John S. Haller, Jr., and Robin M. Haller, *The Physician and Sexuality in Victorian America* (Urbana, 1974), and Ronald Walters, *Primers for Prudery* (New York, 1974). The idea of repression has been especially influential in the concept of "separate spheres" for men and women. See Barbara Welter, "The Cult of True Womanhood," *American Quarterly* (1966) and G. J. Barker-Benfield, *The Horrors of the Half-Known Life: Male Attitudes Toward Women and Sexuality in Nineteenth-Century America* (New York, 1976). Other works that stress separate spheres are two articles in *Signs*: Nancy Cott, "Passionlessness: An Interpretation of Victorian Sexual Ideology" (1978), and Carol Smith Rosenberg, "The Female World of Love and Ritual" (1975).

Carl Degler's "What Ought to Be and What Was," *American Historical Review* (1974) argued that in Victorian morality there was a distinct difference between a repressive ideology and actual behavior. This point is developed further in his *At Odds: Women and the Family in America from the Revolution to the Present* (New York, 1980), and in Peter Gay, *Education of the Senses*, vol. 1, *The Bourgeois Experience: Victoria to Freud* (New York, 1984). The "repressive hypothesis" is further challenged by Ellen K. Rothman, *Hands and Hearts: A History of Courtship in America* (New York, 1985). And it collapses totally in Karen Lystra's major reevaluation of the literature, *Searching the Heart: Women, Men, and Romantic Love in Nineteenth-Century America* (New York, 1989), which illuminates fully the world of "romantic love" in courtship. Works which perhaps exaggerate the extent to which Victorians were not repressed include Patricia Anderson, *When Passion Reigned* (New York, 1995), and Carol Zisowitz Stearns and Peter Stearns, "Victorian Sexuality: Can Historians Do It Better?," *Journal of Social History* (1985). An important case for a functional Victorian morality has been made by Charles Rosenberg, "Sexuality, Class, and Social Role in Nineteenth-Century America," *American Quarterly* (1973).

The importance of the Victorian underworld has yet to be fully understood and integrated into the literature. There is much dependence on British works such as Kellow Chesney's *The Anti-Society: An Account of the Victorian Underworld* (Boston, 1970), or on Steven Marcus's literary study *The Other Victorians* (New York, 1966). Elliott Gorn, *The Manly Art: Bare-Knuckle Prize Fighting in America* (Ithaca, 1986) offers us a glimpse into this world. But it is better developed in Timothy Gilfoyle, *City of Eros: New York City, Prostitution, and the Commercialization of Sex, 1790–1920* (New York, 1992). As we might expect, there is much work on prostitution, notably Neil Shumsky, "Tacit Acceptance: Respectable Americans and Segregated Prostitution, 1870–1910," *Journal of Social History* (1986). The significance of the underworld for Victorian morality is fully integrated in Gertrude Himmelfarb's *The De-moralization of Society: From Victorian Virtues to Modern Values* (New York, 1994), which appreciates the importance of the "self-induced morality, the internalized conscience" at the core of Victorian morality. John Kasson, in *Rudeness & Civility* (New York, 1991), captures brilliantly the ambiguity of Victorian morality. Howard Chudacoff, *The Age of the Bachelor* (1999) sheds new light on the transition to the twentieth century.

THE PROGRESSIVE ERA REVOLUTION

The breaching of the conspiracy of silence was first identified in a classic article by John Burnham, "The Progressive Era Revolution in American Attitudes Towards Sex," *Journal of American History* (1973). Numerous scholars have examined the Greenwich Village bohemians. Especially valuable are William L. O'Neill's *Divorce in the Progressive Era* (New Haven, 1967) and Christopher Lasch, *The New Radicalism in America, 1889–1963* (New York, 1965). But Edward Abrahams, *The Lyrical Left* (Charlottesville, Va., 1984) offers a more recent critique. Leslie Fishbein, *Rebels in Bohemia* (Chapel Hill, 1982) is a useful introduction to the scene.

James McGovern first identified the extent of women's growing freedom before World War I in "The American Woman's Pre–World War One Freedom in Manners and Morals," *Journal of American History* (1968). But most work on women in the period has focused on the working class: Kathy Peiss, *Cheap Amusements: Working Women and Leisure in Turn-of-the-Century New York* (Philadelphia, 1986) on New York, and Joanne Meyerowitz, *Women Adrift* (Chicago, 1988) on Chicago. The pioneer in studies of turn-of-the-century leisure was John Kasson, *Amusing the Million: Coney Island at the Turn of the Century* (New York, 1978).

On birth control, David Kennedy, *Birth Control in America:*

The Career of Margaret Sanger (New York, 1970) remains a standard work. But the importance of Mary Ware Dennett has recently been recognized in Constance C. Chen, *The Sex Side of Life* (New York, 1996). On the war campaigns, the definitive work is Allan Brandt, *No Magic Bullet: A Social History of Venereal Disease in the United States Since 1880* (New York, 1985), which tries to place the early period in the context of the contemporary AIDS crisis.

THE 1920S AND 1930S

The idea that the 1920s saw a revolution in morals has been a standard trope in American history since Frederick Lewis Allen's classic journalistic survey *Only Yesterday: An Informal History of the 1920s* (New York, 1931). His ideas were picked up by William Leuchtenburg in *The Perils of Prosperity, 1914–32* (New York, 1957) and in George Mowry, *The Urban Nation, 1920–1960* (New York, 1965). The "flapper" phenomenon was brilliantly diagnosed by Kenneth Yellis in "Prosperity's Child: Some Thoughts on the Flapper," *American Quarterly* (1969). Since the 1970s, feminist criticism of the stereotypical and male-defined picture of women that she represented has abounded. This began with Estelle Freedman, "The New Woman," *Journal of American History* (1974), and was aggressively developed by Nancy Cott in *The Grounding of Modern Feminism* (New Haven, 1987), which confirms the origins of increased women's sexual demands in these years for birth control and for abortion. A moving account of the dilemmas faced by one leading feminist is Leila J. Rupp's skillful "Feminism and the Sexual Revolution of the Early Twentieth Century: The Case of Doris Stevens," *Feminist Studies* (1989). The male experience of the revolution is addressed in Kevin White's *The First Sexual Revolution: The Emergence of Male Heterosexuality in Modern America* (New York, 1993).

Aspects of this revolution have been well studied. Lary May's *Screening Out the Past* (New York, 1980) is excellent on the movies. Mae West receives her due in Marybeth Hamilton's *When I'm Bad, I'm Better* (New York, 1996). On the moral code, see Gregory D. Black, *Hollywood Censored: Morality Codes, Catholics, and the Movies* (Cambridge, Mass., 1994). On literature, Frederick Hoffman, *The Twenties: American Writing in the Postwar Decade* (New York, 1955) remains definitive. Advertising has been covered in Roland Marchand's *Advertising the American Dream* (New York, 1985), and less satisfactorily in T. J. Jackson Lears's *Fables of Abundance: A Cultural History of Advertising in America* (New York, 1994). An excellent article on sex and marriage manuals is Peter Laipson, "Kiss Without Shame for She Deserves It," *Journal of Social History* (1996). On the Harlem Renaissance, see David Levering Lewis, *When Harlem Was in Vogue* (New York, 1993). On divorce, see Elaine Tyler May, *Great Expectations: Marriage and Divorce in Post-Victorian America* (Chicago, 1980).

Absolutely indispensable for all historians of the period between the wars is Robert and Helen Lynd, *Middletown* and *Middletown in Transition* (New York, 1929, 1937), the pioneering sociological surveys of Muncie, Indiana.

While it is agreed that there was something different about the 1920s, the complexity of the changes are recognized (and the appropriateness of such terms as "revolution in morals" and "sexual revolution" are being questioned). Most valuable are Christina Simmons, "The Myth of Victorian Repression," in Simmons and Kathy Peiss, eds., *Passion and Power* (Baltimore, 1989), and Kevin White, "The New Man and Early Twentieth Century Emotional Culture," in Peter Stearns and Jan Lewis, eds., *An Emotional History of the United States* (New York, 1998).

The depression's impact on sexuality and the family has been neglected. The most thorough exploration is the chapter in John Modell's *Into One's Own* (Berkeley, 1989), or in Steven Mintz and Susan Kellogg, *Domestic Revolutions*. John C. Spurlock and Cynthia Magistro's *New and Improved: The Transformation of American Women's Emotional Culture* (New York, 1998) gives much attention to the depression. Otherwise we must depend on primary source material such as that by the Chicago sociologists, such as Paul Cressey, *The Taxi-Dance Hall* (Chicago, 1932), or the early sex survey by Lewis Terman, *Psychological Factors in Marital Happiness* (New York, 1938).

THE 1950S

The impact of World War II on sexual attitudes is covered in Beth Bailey and David Farber's *The First Strange Place: The Alchemy of Race and Sex in World War II Hawaii* (New York, 1993). David Reynolds, *Rich Relations: The American Occupation of Britain, 1942–1945* (New York, 1995) is an excellent source on the mores of the American occupying forces. Allan Bérubé, *Coming Out Under Fire* (New York, 1990) discusses the formation of gay identity in the war.

The attack on Kinsey grows apace, so that his reputation is now in free fall. James H. Jones, *Alfred C. Kinsey: A Public/Private Life* (New York, 1997) convincingly deflates him. It is unlikely that Kinsey will be rehabilitated by Jonathan Gathorne-Hardy, *Sex, the Measure of All Things: A Life of Alfred C. Kinsey* (London, 1998), which tries to defend him.

The view of the 1950s as a revival of Victorian values is stubbornly adhered to in William L. O'Neill's *American High* (New York, 1986). Elaine Tyler May, in *Homeward Bound: American Families in the Cold War Era* (Chicago, 1989), basically agrees with O'Neill but sees the return of family values as a bad thing, the result of Cold War mobilization. She relies heavily on Betty Friedan's rather spurious interpretation in *The Feminine Mystique* (New York, 1963), which in turn influenced Barbara Ehrenreich's *The Hearts of Men: American Dreams and the Flight from Commitment* (New York, 1983). Wini Breines's *Young, White, and Miserable* (New York, 1994) offers a compelling and personalized account of how sexual repression for women allegedly linked up with repression of African Americans. The problems faced by pregnant unmarried women are explored by Rickie Solinger in *Wake Up Little Susie: Single Pregnancy Before Roe v. Wade* (New York, 1994).

The implications for sexual morality of rock music have not received the attention the subject deserves. I have relied heavily on Ed Ward, et al., *Rock of Ages: The Rolling Stone History of Rock & Roll* (New York, 1986). The first serious work to look at gender and rock is Joy Press and Simon Reynolds, *The Sex Revolts* (London, 1995). Work on Elvis Presley is voluminous but largely worthless. Albert Goldman's biography *Elvis* (New York, 1981) is disturbing and lacks empathy. Peter Guralnick's *Last Train to Memphis* (1991) and *Careless Love: The Unmaking of Elvis Presley* (1999) are useful.

The Beats have inspired much writing. The best history is Michael Davidson, *The Beat Generation* (San Francisco, 1989). See also Ann Charters, *Kerouac* (New York, 1973), and Barry Miles, *Ginsberg* (New York, 1989). On gays in the 1950s, John D'Emilio, *Sexual Politics, Sexual Communities: The Making of a Homosexual Minority in the United States, 1940–1970* (Chicago, 1983) is the standard work and is likely to remain so for some time to come.

THE 1960S AND 1970S

Very little historical work has appeared on the sexual revolution of this period. Beth Bailey, *Sex in the Heartland* (Cambridge, Mass., 1999) is a start. Much of the chaos was understood by William L. O'Neill in *Coming Apart: An Informal History of America in the 1960s* (New York, 1971). We depend on such contemporary works as Vance Packard's *The Sexual Wilderness* (New York, 1968), or Helen Gurley Brown's *Sex and the Single Girl* (New York, 1963). An excellent account of the shenanigans of a rock group in America (the Kinks) is Ray Davies's *X-Ray* (London, 1995). On the Doors, see Daniel Sugerman and Jerry Hopkins, *No One Here Gets Out Alive* (New York, 1981).

On the Pill, see Patrick Allitt, *Catholic Intellectuals and Conservative Politics in America, 1950–1985* (Ithaca, 1993) and Beth Bailey, "Prescribing the Pill," *Journal of Social History* (1997). Barbara Ehrenreich, *Re-Making Love* (New York, 1986), and

218   A NOTE ON SOURCES

Linda Grant, *Sexing the Millennium* (New York, 1994) offer useful information and insights.

The history of the modern women's movement is now beginning to be written. Radical feminism has so far elicited the most
attention. Sara Evans, *Personal Politics* (New York, 1978) was an
early effort by a participant to analyze women's experience in the
civil rights movement. Alice Echols, *Daring to Be Bad: Radical
Feminism in America, 1967–1975* (Minneapolis, 1989) will be the
definitive history of radical feminism in its period for a long time
to come. On gay rights, Martin Duberman, *Stonewall* (New
York, 1994) is a moving account of the riots. Edmund White,
States of Desire: Travels in Gay America (New York, 1980) is a
wonderful account of gay life in the period.

           1980 TO THE PRESENT

Here we move from the province of the historian to that of the
sociologist and cultural critic. The AIDS crisis has generated an
enormous amount of material. The definitive account of the
early epidemic is Randy Shilts, *And the Band Played On* (New
York, 1987). Early sociological perspectives were provided by
Cindy Patton, *Sex and Germs* (New York, 1986), and Dennis Altman, *AIDS in the Mind of America* (Boston, 1985).

The anxieties that traditionalists feel over illegitimacy and
shifting mores are expressed in Charles Murray and Richard
Herrnstein, *Losing Ground: American Social Policy, 1950–1980*
(New York, 1984) and *The Bell Curve: Intelligence and Class
Structure in American Life* (New York, 1994).

Sex surveys have been voluminous. The Hite Reports that
began in 1975 have been a source of amusement. Two recent sex
surveys are more deserving of attention: Lillian Rubin's *Erotic
Wars: What Happened to the Sexual Revolution?* (New York,
1991), and Robert T. Michael, et al., *Sex in America* (Boston,
1994).

In the 1980s, feminism continued to be in ascendancy as an

ideology, despite the unsympathetic Reagan presidency. But by the 1990s the women's movement was experiencing a barrage of criticism from within, notably from Christina Hoff Sommers, *Who Stole Feminism? How Women Have Betrayed Women* (New York, 1994); Elizabeth Fox-Genovese, *Feminism Without Illusions* (Chapel Hill, 1991); and, most petulantly, Katie Roiphe, *The Morning After* (New York, 1993). A couple of younger writers have tried to restore credibility to the women's movement, notably Susan Faludi's earnest *Backlash: The Undeclared War Against Women* (New York, 1991), and Naomi Wolf's *Fire with Fire* (New York, 1993). Feminists found it hard to answer legitimate accusations of political correctness that exposed the privileged's efforts to stifle the expression of the underprivileged. Richard Bernstein's *Dictatorship of Virtue: Multiculturalism and the Battle for America's Future* (New York, 1994), and Robert Hughes's *The Culture of Complaint: The Fraying of America* (New York, 1993) contributed to the debate over political correctness, which necessarily involved feminists.

On Clinton's America, David Blankenhorn's *Fatherless America* (New York, 1996), Dana Mack's *The Assault on Parenthood: How Our Culture Undermines the Family* (New York, 1997), and Barbara DaFoe Whitehead's *The Divorce Culture* (New York, 1996) are three particularly compelling attacks that seem to prefigure and predict the moral rot at the top in these years. But they pale in comparison with Robert Bork's olympian *Slouching Towards Gomorrah* (New York, 1996).

Gay America hasn't just been about AIDS, especially in the 1990s. Carrying on in a tradition started by Seymour Kleinberg's *Alienated Affections: Being Gay in America* (New York, 1980), Bruce Bawer's *A Place at the Table* (New York, 1994) pleads the gay case for mainstream acceptance. So does Andrew Sullivan's *Virtually Normal: An Argument About Homosexuality* (New York, 1995).

Robert Bly's *Iron John* (New York, 1990) convincingly suggests that men have lost out since the sexual revolution. The best book on the men's movement is Michael Schwalbe's *Unlocking the Iron Cage: The Men's Movement, Gender Politics, and American Culture* (New York, 1996).

An effort to address the future is Katie Roiphe, *Last Night in Paradise: Sex and Morals at the Century's End* (New York, 1997), while an interesting but nostalgic turn-of-the-millennium effort to recapture the flavor of Victorianism is Wendy Shalit, *A Return to Modesty: Discovering the Lost Virtue* (New York, 1999).

Index

Internet, 208
Intolerance (Griffith), 46–47
Irwin, Will, 25
Israels, Belle Lindner, 44

Jackson, Michael, 185, 204
Jackson, Millie, 180
Jagger, Mick, 177
James, Harry, 98
Jones, James H., 112
Jones, Landon, 106
Jones, Paula, 207
Jong, Erica, 158
Joy of Sex, The (Comfort), 150
Joyce, James, 83
Juvenile delinquency in 1950s,
    121, 123

Kaiser Family Foundation, 206
Kameny, Franklin, 166–167
Kantner, John F., 151
Karalus, Charlaine, 113
Katz, Jonathan, 72
Kazan, Elia, 122
Kemp, Harry, 63, 64
Kennedy, Elizabeth, 132
Kennedy, John F., 162
Kennedy, Ted, 171
Kent, Samuel, 72
Kerouac, Jack, 126–127
Key, Ellen, 29–30
"Khaki Wackies," 102

Khrushchev, Nikita, 109
Kimmel, Michael, 200
King, Carole, 145
Kinks, 177
Kinsey, Alfred Charles, 77,
    110–112, 131, 149, 195; on
    abortions, 93; on homosexual-
    ity, 111, 130, 196; on infidelity
    during World War II, 102;
    James H. Jones on, 112; on
    men, 111; 1960s and living
    dream of, 134; on women, 111
Kinsey Institute on gays, 173
Kleinschmidt, H. E., 51
Koedt, Ann, 160
Komarovsky, Mirra, 91
Kopay, Dave, 171
Koss, Mary, 190
Kramer, Larry, 173, 193
Kramer, Stanley, 121
Kruth, Joseph Wood, 86
Kubrick, Stanley, 139–140, 175

La Dolce Vita, 139
LaBelle, Patti, 180
Landis, Paul, 108
Lange, Jessica, 188
Lasch, Christopher, 33
Lawrence, D. H., 136
Lawrence, Steve, 146
Le Sueur, Meridel, 91, 92
Lee, Spike, 188
Legion of Decency, 85, 141
Lennox, Annie, 184